Revealing Your Inner Radiance:

HEALING THROUGH THE HEART

Dr. Christina Tarantola, PharmD, CHC

Copyright © 2015 by Christina Tarantola

Edited by Michelle Josette
www.mjbookeditor.com

Thank you Mom and Dad, for your generosity, discipline and love, but most of all for giving me the lessons I needed.

I also want to thank my mentor, Dr. Sweta Chawla, who showed me unconditional love, showed me how to open my heart. She was my spiritual soul-mate and guide through this journey.

I am so grateful for Aunt Grace, Ellen, Tonya, Justin, Gerald, Tatiana, Phil, and all of the people who supported me in my endeavors. I am so grateful for you.

Thanks to all of the women and coaches from Mastin Kipp's Daily Love Mastermind. Without you all, this book would not be what it is today.

Dr Chawla,

"And when you want something, all the universe conspires in helping you achieve it". - The Alchemist

There will be endless gratitude for you for being the strongest person in my weakest moments.

With Love,

Ch

Preface

"Each one of us, regardless of our situation, is looking for the same treasure in the ashes. We are in search of our most authentic, vital, generous and wise self. What stands between that self and us is what burns in the fire. Our illusions, our rigidity, our fear, our blame and our sense of separation: All of these—in varying strengths and combinations—are what must die in order for a more true self to arise. The great loneliness—like the loneliness a caterpillar endures when she wraps herself in a silky shroud and begins the long transformation from chrysalis to butterfly. It seems that we too must go through such a time, when life as we know it is over—when being a caterpillar feels somehow false and yet we don't know who we are supposed to become. All we know is that something bigger is calling us to change. And though we must make the journey alone, and even if suffering is our only companion, soon enough we will become a butterfly, soon enough we will taste the rapture of being alive." *Broken Open: How Difficult Times Can Help Us Grow* | Elizabeth Lesser

The healing journey is one of extreme courage. The word "courage" comes from the Latin word *cour* meaning heart. Only the brave of heart have the strength to take the journey to bring awareness and light to the darkest parts of themselves, to perform an emotional alchemy and to reemerge transformed.

An integral part of healing comes from connecting with your heart and breaking free of the ego-mind. This is why ancient sages took retreats for days of silence and why transcendental meditation and deep-breathing exercises are revered for stress relief and relaxation. When you detach from the ego-mind, you remove all ego and situations—things people have said or done no longer matter. Love is the elixir for all problems, barriers, and disputes. And the heart is where love pours out in insurmountable quantities.

Loving yourself unconditionally is the number one priority to healing any disease, rejection of the self, disorder or malignancy. Why is self-love so important and integral to healing? When you resist yourself, or the true nature of who you are, you cause more stress and place your attention on negative thoughts regarding the illness/disease. Developing and cultivating your sense of personal power and self-love is like the foundation of your house. Something magnificent cannot be built on a turbulent or weakened structure.

Your self-love will never abandon you, deny, or deprive you. It is your core essence, your foundation, your holiness. Your self-love will be the only thing that will get you up to feed the kids and go to work after you feel frustrated, hopeless, and tired after you've binged through an entire bag of chips or a pint of ice cream. It will be there after you've been feared, guilted, and coerced by the misshapen definition of someone else's conditional love for you. It will ground you. It will be there when your spirit is so broken and you've got nothing left but the clothes on your back and a prayer in your heart to keep you going.

You see, no one can give that love to you. No one can give you what you do not already possess for yourself. Yet as humans, we seek love externally to feel worthy, to feel that we are "enough." Your entire life may have been based upon chasing a feeling or a core set of feelings—love, approval, attention, belonging. You may be a seeker like I was, never really understanding why you have an underlying unhappiness, unease, and discomfort through everyday life. I am here to show you that when you are in alignment—in congruence with your deepest desires and values and you act, think, and speak those desires—you are in integrity. This is the place of health, vitality, and boundless energy!

Yet so many of us construct our lives around feeling safe and secure in our jobs, relationships and finances, and thus our personal integrity is compromised. Those feelings of certainty are shallow and fleeting, allowing us to think there is something else "out there" to satiate the hunger that burns in our bellies. What happens if we rely on the security of our husband/wife for our identity and suddenly they divorce us or the marriage subtly unzips at the seams, leaving us emotionally deprived? What would happen if our job was no longer there to provide that feeling of safety and security? We go to the next best thing that will provide security and safety—food, alcohol, cigarettes, or some other external "thing."

We do this because those things give us a *feeling*. It is not the physical quality alone that keeps us addicted and continues the vicious cycle; it is the psychological certainty and safety we crave that temporarily fills these voids. Once this cycle begins, it is difficult to break. In my experience with food addiction, it was like a torrid love affair. Each night I would wake up for my next 'fix' ready to consume, to numb, to feel certain I was safe.

I was numbing myself and hiding who I was, shameful to show my essence, my radiance, my true colors. It took me 7 years and a plethora of therapists, mentors, guides, self-help books, and dozens of sleepless nights to gain the awareness I have now. Who was I to be great, to shine in the world and make a difference? Who was I to be happy, energetic and full of life? I didn't feel safe enough to escape an environment where I was constantly criticized and shamed. I was not fully expressing all of my talents, my unique gifts, touching people around me like I needed to, like my soul was calling me to do. I NEEDED to connect meaningfully with people. Yet I was so held back by my past and the belief of "not being good enough," and was thus creating that reality of lack around me. I did not have deep, meaningful relationships, and I used food to feel full because I always felt empty.

The only way out was through—I knew and understood after years of mentally exhausting myself, physically abusing my body by waking up every single night and eating. I developed 12 cavities because of it. But my self-love pushed me through. It always pushed me through. Even though I only had a glimpse of it, a teaspoonful, it was enough to spark a huge transformation and change my life forever. It was time for me to wake up to my inner radiance…

Introduction

This book is meant to serve as a guide for anyone who is a seeker to understand and utilize different modalities of healing, or purely to see the world through a new lens. I was a seeker for many years and could not understand my disease. The concept of disease as I will mention later in this book, is caused by being disconnected from yourself in some aspect. You have forgotten or lost some part of yourself, which has created a breach in your energy field (physical, mental/emotional, or spiritual.) Along my journey, I stumbled, fell down and got back up just to be challenged again and again. I have such a deep level of respect for you and your journey because it is unique and not always easy to travel down.

A series of destiny-shaping events sparked my passion to create this book. I was suffering with a rare eating disorder, having daily bouts of anxiety, low energy, and toxic, depleting relationships. When I was at my rock-bottom, I prayed for a miracle to be healed. I promised myself that if I did heal, I would share my story and the *how* of my way out of that Dark Night of the Soul.

I believe there is a *message* and a *mission* within you, and you can feel frustrated and empty when you are not expressing those two things in the world. Your tests become your testimony and that message is simply your road to awakening who you really are. This is coming back home to yourself. This is true healing. The mission is what you take from that message and the guided action steps that produce the greatest fulfillment you will ever know. This is my intention for you—that you discover and reveal your authentic message and mission through reading my story.

I have divided my book into two parts. Part I is taken from specific and relevant events in my life and my personal healing journey. I want to tell this story to show you that any disease can be healed. You may be saying, *Wow, what a loaded statement! What if someone has terminal cancer, a life-threatening illness, or is on their death bed?* Healing can still occur on a person's death bed. If a person has breath, they can participate in their own healing.

Healing occurs on many levels—spiritual, mental/emotional, and physical. I would like to be your guide to help you ease and eradicate any pain you have. My intention is for you to close this book and know more about yourself, to gain more energy, and to have a greater appreciation for life and the people who fill it.

I believe we all have the power of choice and awareness, most of which shape our lives. I also believe that inside each of us is a beautiful, pure, core essence. We are all born with unique gifts, talents, and a soul-mission. As you grow, fears from family and others around you cause you to absorb those fears and forget the pure radiance that is always available to you. Fear causes pain, but love heals wounds. I made a clear decision to craft my life the way I would like it to be when it was too much to bear, when I wanted to give up on myself. I believe the same is possible for you. You can literally create and design your life how YOU would like it to be. All it takes is courage to walk through the fears and the pain in order to emerge as your radiant self. This is who you have always been.

At the beginning of 2014, I declared that I wanted to laugh and connect with strangers, move into a home where I felt comfortable and connected to the culture around me, and fulfill my dream of writing this book. Within a month I had moved from my isolated apartment in Howard Beach to Brooklyn and had received an email from Mastin Kipp from the Daily Love with an offer to interview. I would be attending his retreat and writing my story in Bali. I took a leap of faith and signed up for The Daily Love Writers Mastermind group that would take place in November of 2014. As things began shifting in my life, I realized how the universe worked with me to co-create the possibilities I so deeply desired. I embarked on a journey of a lifetime, going to Bali with Mastin and my new family of 29 other writers. With their support, I wrote this book. I knew I needed to tell the story of my own healing journey to set the stage for Part II: Healing Through the Heart.

In addition, Part II has "prescriptions" for healing and health at the end of each chapter. These tools are a culmination of all that I have come to learn about health, the disease process, and various modalities of healing.

I am asking you, before you read another sentence, to commit to doing the exercises in Part II. If you decide to close this book now and put it back on the shelf, I completely understand. But I also want to ask you, are you the type of person who has said, "I've tried EVERYTHING!" If you are and you have felt angry, frustrated, stuck, and confused in any area of your life, please stay with me.

You may see yourself in my story or the countless stories I speak about with the patients and clients I have seen. It is my greatest intention that you receive the highest good from these amazing souls whom I have come across. I am grateful you came across this book—that the universe decided it was destined to fall into your lap.

Peace and love,
Christina

Part I

Chapter 1: It's a Beautiful Life

I believe there are many days in a person's life that are poignant, memorable, and thrilling. Some may be filled with joy, such as the day a parent witnesses the birth of their first child. That innocence of seeing a newborn open its tiny eyes can bring even the most stoic of men to tears of joy. Or perhaps such feelings may be expressed the day a father walks his daughter down the aisle to be given away to the man she will spend the rest of her life with. It is the feeling of pure elation that makes those moments stick in our minds forever.

However, the scariest, most uncertain day of a person's life may be the day they are diagnosed with a life-threatening illness. Life becomes very real and precious in that moment. When the words "cancer" or "diabetes" or "tumor" are spoken from a doctor's mouth, a human life is changed in an instant. Those moments are just as poignant, however they fully grip fear, doubt, pain, and anger and look it straight in the face. Those spoken words ring in someone's ears for days, weeks, and months to follow. They may involve family, friends, doctors, and dozens of other people, and can stick in a person's mind forever.

Disease, or a lack of harmony and balance in the body, manifests in many ways—from pain, headaches, anxiety, depression, fatigue, and acne, all the way to cancer. And we are all susceptible to it. There are many physical causes of disease as modern science has studied and documented. Smoking, excess consumption of animal meat and alcohol, lack of exercise, and both mental and physical stress are some causes, to name a few. Researchers have spent copious amounts of time and money to draw massive cohorts of people together to study, research, and document patterns of behavior, how the body responds to stress, and how to prevent and treat disease. Much of this research has helped create treatment algorithms that medical doctors now implement.

As a pharmacist, I have personally witnessed the miraculous workings of pharmaceuticals, which rescue millions of lives each year. Antiarrhythmic drugs help reestablish normal heart rhythms in patients with atrial fibrillation. Emergency-room doctors administer vasopressor, epinephrine, and other blood pressure stabilizers that literally save people's lives. I have also seen thousands of patients on opioids, mood-stabilizing medications, amphetamines, and appetite suppressants. These controlled substances leave a person tolerant, needing higher doses to achieve the same effect over time. Even many people on blood pressure medication were not satisfied with the adverse effects of their medications and wanted alternative answers. However, most medication is a Catch-22, a double-edged sword. First, you are only treating the "symptoms" and never getting to the root "cause." In addition, your body is succumbed to a multitude of adverse effects including vitamin depletion, and begins to rely on the medication to function.

As I began my work as a pharmacist, I became intimately involved with talking to patients about their experiences with medication as it related to their health condition. As I mentioned, most of them did not want to be on medication; they wanted a natural therapy. Many of them took vitamins, supplements, and over-the-counter products. They often asked their friends about their health conditions or even searched their symptoms on the Internet before going to a doctor. People wanted to feel better, to alleviate pain or lose weight or lower their blood pressure through natural means. That was the point when I realized that understanding pharmaceuticals alone would not serve my patients. I began learning more about alternative medicine, the healing benefits of food, and eventually energy healing and Applied Kinesiology.

In pharmacy school, I learned about the inner workings of biological pathways, how the body functioned normally and how the disease process occurred. Pathology, or the study of the cause and effect of disease, made sense at the time. In order to function normally, each system of the body has to stay in equilibrium with the organ, tissues, and cells associated. Any disruption in the system caused inflammation or an imbalance of some sort that could be corrected with a drug.

Most of the classes of medications we learned started with *anti*, or "against life." Anti-inflammatory, antidepressant, antipsychotic, antiseptic…these drugs worked against the body, however they synthetically regulated the system to equilibrate back to normal functioning.

In my Drugs and Disease courses, I studied how drugs were absorbed, metabolized, distributed into different tissues to exert their mechanism, and how they were eliminated from the body. Each drug had a unique mechanism to target a receptor for a certain amount of time and was then eliminated by the kidney, skin, lungs, or liver. But the drug would only last so long in the body (also known as its "half-life") and another dose was needed.

In addition side effects resulted from the medication since each drug is a xenobiotic—a synthetic foreign substance. We were taught to counsel our patients on how to minimize those side effects by taking the pill at night if it caused drowsiness or taking a diuretic early in the morning to prevent a nighttime run to the bathroom. So many questions were left unanswered.

In the case of an illness that had no tangible origin like depression, anxiety, or an eating disorder, the explanation was vague and lacking in evidence. Was it enough to say the cause was genetic or an amalgamation of environmental factors like abuse and stress? Why did certain people heal but others did not? It made sense that in the case of heart disease, for example, poor diet, lack of exercise, or continuous smoking led to plaque buildup in the arteries known as atherosclerosis, and eventually led to a heart attack or stroke. I had so many questions buzzing through my mind, and they would remain unanswered until I began to understand my own disease as well as energy work.

Because of my own eating disorder and seeing so many sick patients coming back to the pharmacy month after month for refills and never improving, I became obsessed with understanding *why* people got sick and how they could *heal*. I searched for the answers in self-help books, sought out reading material from mind-body-medicine gurus like Dr. Deepak Chopra and Dr. Andrew Weil. Some of the most significant findings I came across were those of Barbara Brennan, who studied the tenets of energy healing, and Dr. David Hawkins, who studied Applied Kinesiology (AK) and calibrated the Energy Vibration Scale after 20 years of research.

Hawkins' research drew upon thousands of people over several decades to study kinesiology, how the body responded to false and true beliefs. He studied Electromagnetic Frequency (EMF), outlining a consciousness scale ranging from 0 to 1000. False statements or harmful substances would weaken the person's muscles and lead to a strong emotional "No" reaction, whereas when a person held a life-promoting substance or spoke a true statement, a clear "Yes" would come across. Low vibrational thoughts such as guilt, shame, and fear kept people in a contracted, limited state, while love, joy, and gratitude led them to align with health and happiness.

These concepts were in strong correlation with the patterns I began noticing with my patients. I saw many clients with diabetes and eating disorders, but the conversation was rarely just about food. Feelings of self-hatred, guilt, shame, anger, unwillingness to forgive, frustration, and other heavy emotions would surface as we worked through why they overate or tried to control their food. I realized then that people had certain energy blockages that prevented them from being fully radiant, energetic, and healthy.

Of note, it has been documented that many people with eating disorders such as compulsive overeaters usually had a painful trauma that caused them tremendous pain in childhood (rape or sexual abuse, death of a loved one, job or marital issues, or unresolved issues such as emotional abandonment from a parent). This leads them to overeat and connect with food instead of forming healthy connections with themselves and other people. In my focus group for eating disorder treatment, I noticed those people had the same patterns. My heart felt for every one of my clients and even some close friends. I knew that suffering myself and wanted desperately to help them out of it. So I kept researching…

After studying Barbara Brennan's work on energy healing, I marveled at the ideas she spoke about. She reasons that most diseases stem from a disconnection with source and with self. In essence, if a person is not living in truth with their deepest desires and connected to a divine source, they will suffer. If that spiritual level is not aligned then that disruption in their energy field fans out to toxic thoughts/feelings and finally manifests into physical symptoms. I knew how people stayed "well" by using prescription drugs that kept them normalized chemically, but how did someone *heal?*

In order to determine the real cause of disease and to heal, you have to go to the root, which is in essence a spiritual problem. If you are sick, it means you have forgotten some aspect of who you really are. Somewhere along the way you have compromised your truth or your will. Please do not take me saying this as judgment or punishment that you deserve this disease. I fully believe you are meant to be healthy and happy, and I am committed to help guide you toward revealing the essence of who you really are.

It will take some work! After all, I am sure that if you are frustrated it is for a good reason. You may have tried several healing modalities already, which have led you to this moment. You may have even said, "I've tried EVERYTHING!" I commend you because I know what it's like to go searching for answers, and I pray that you will feel better.

Tony Robbins said, "The destiny of your life lies in your ability to deal with massive uncertainty." So much of our patterns are certain and familiar and they pacify us yet keep us stuck all at once.

Stepping into uncertainty — out of your comfort zone, even just a little — can cause a massive shift and a breakthrough for your health and happiness. I am asking you to trust me that if you stick with it, even when you get frustrated, you will begin to heal.

The process of digging through your past to understand why you have this disease will guide you toward reveal your inner radiance — your healthy, vibrant self. This takes a bit of time and energy, but when it is complete, you will feel incredible, filled with joy and aligned with health.

Picture a nagging weed that keeps growing in your garden. Naturally, you would want to pull it out so it doesn't shroud the light for the other flowers. I used to weed the garden with my mother growing up. I was assigned the task of pulling out dandelions. (Go figure, dandelions can actually be used for liver detoxification!) My mother taught me that you cannot just pull at the leaves or the stems; you need to get to the root of the weed to effectively pull it out. If you just break the stalk, the root is still there and the weed will grow again. The same goes for disease. Many people pull at the stalk, yank at the dandelion flower but never get to the root cause. They mask symptoms by taking prescription drugs or anesthetizing themselves with alcohol or food.

As I began to make sense of the cause of disease, I realized the same schematic that leads to disease is also the pathway to healing. Embedded within each layer of the PEMS (Physical, Emotional/Mental, Spiritual), you may have certain feelings and ask certain questions. Each layer can be described as follows:

Spiritual Layer

- Feelings: Hopelessness, Feeling lost
- Questions: Where do I belong? What is my purpose? Do people understand me?

Mental/Emotional Layer

- Manifestation: Confusion, Despair, Migraines
- Feelings: Grief, Depression, Anxiety, Fear, Apathy, Confusion, Frustration, Heaviness, Worthlessness, Unsupported
- Questions: What is the point? What will become of me?

Physical Layer

- Manifestation: Weight gain, Acne, Headache/migraine, Chronic Pain, Fatigue/Lethargy
- Feelings: Shame, Guilt
- Questions: Why is this happening? Why do I have to suffer?

If you are like me, you may be asking these questions now or have asked them in the past. Where do I get help? Do I go to a traditional doctor, a naturopath, an herbalist, or an acupuncturist? Do I self-treat? Ignore the problem? If you are reading this book now, you have already taken one step closer to healing. You are showing willingness that most people do not want to face — to decide that they are fed up with the old ways of behaving and not taking care of their body, mind, and soul. It takes courage to come on this journey, and it is worth every step of the way. I fully support you.

I can tell you that if you take an honest look at what you have been avoiding or denying about yourself, you will heal. If you take an honest inventory of where you have not been speaking your truth or living in integrity, you will heal. If you can be willing and vulnerable enough to admit your beautiful imperfections and cultivate self-love, you will align with health. This is the power of personal transformation.

The pathway to the root cause of disease is also the pathway to healing. Alignment of PEMS is the gateway to health. If a person has acne, there can be dietary factors that exacerbate the condition. Acne is a disruption in the *physical field* and can usually be traced back through the chakra system to the first chakra. When examined with curiosity, there may be feelings that the person does not feel supported by life and does not feel comfortable in their own skin. There may be thoughts/feelings of unworthiness, suppressed anger, insecurity, and lack of support in the Mental/Emotional layer. Acne and other skin conditions, lower back pain, constipation, and most other first-chakra imbalances can be healed by connecting with the self through meditation, and redirecting your thoughts to more positive ones so you feel connected to the people around you.

I will tell you this with confidence: You know how to heal yourself. Yes, doctors are there to listen, assess, diagnose, and treat illness. Yes, they absolutely save lives. Yet an autonomy exists as well as a physician-patient relationship that allows you to decide *with* the doctor, naturopath, or whatever practitioner you see. *You* have the inner guidance to know if you should try Reiki healing, aromatherapy, or ask for a second opinion. Always trust your intuition when it comes to your body and your health. Healthcare practitioners are privileged guides to help you heal, but you are the real expert on your own body. All you have to do is trust yourself.

Chapter 2: Hurt so good, come on baby make it hurt so good

The body is a beautiful biological instrument that allows us to perform daily functions and live out our lives. We breathe without thinking about it, our hearts beat in perfect syncope, and blood flows where it is needed. In fact, the body is so intelligent that it knows how to protect you and me. If a person gets cut by a sharp knife and a small wound appears, microscopic white blood cells called macrophages go to the site of injury to repair the wound. Like a small surgical repair, the macrophages stitch up the damage. All of this is perfectly designed, executed, and orchestrated without us having to think about any of it.

It is not so far-fetched, then, to believe the body sends us silent signals all the time. When we are mentally stressed about something, the onset of a headache may appear, or the body may crave something sweet to comfort and soothe us and to increase the mood-boosting chemical serotonin. All of these signals are your body's way of reporting to you that something is off-balance. Something has gone wrong in the system.

Think about it in the case of a plumber. If there is a leak, he goes to the source of the leak to fix it. In the case of a computer repairman, he finds the virus and cleans it out. There is no difference here—your body tries to fix and mend itself by offering you some help and physically showing you what is wrong. The problem is, most of us do not listen to our bodies. Instead we listen to our minds.

Any discomfort in your body is a direct message that you are not in alignment with your true self. This is not a judgment on you or your past. Many concepts I will reveal in this book may resonate with you. Some may cause resistance and make you want to run, avoid that chapter, or close the book all together. My goal for you is to be truthful, honest, and real about how you can feel better. This is coming from me, a person who denied that anything was wrong with me until I got sick.

If you are healthy and were drawn to this book for whatever reason, this content will help prevent you from getting sick and will improve your quality of life. If you are sick or know someone who is, this is the best gift you could give yourself. As you become clearer about what your body really craves by listening to its internal messages, you will come back into balance.

As in Maslow's hierarchy of needs, a human being needs shelter, food, clothing, and water. When you are tired, you need rest. When you are hungry, you need to eat. However, many of us overeat, overwork, and get little sleep. We deprive ourselves of basic needs that all of us need to survive. It sounds so simple, right? *Oh, just listen to your body.* But how do you do that?

First you have to understand the rules of the mind. As human beings we all want to move away from pain and towards pleasure. There is something so appealing about a large movie-sized bag of popcorn that calls to your taste buds. Going on the treadmill for an hour sounds so much less appealing, right? We are wired for pleasure, which is why sex, alcohol, drugs, and entertainment draw huge crowds. We want the quick fix and to avoid feeling our pain because it is so uncomfortable. Yet masking our symptoms and pain with "good feeling" substances is like putting whipped cream on a mud pie. The mud certainly isn't chocolate and even though it looks good from the whipped cream, the deeper layers aren't so tasty!

So, we want to avoid pain, but what is pain? Pain is a nonspecific, or "general," symptom that originates from a variety of different sources. Continuous impact and wear and tear on a joint lead to osteoarthritis. Poor positioning of your desk chair at work can lead to misalignments in the spine and put undue pressure and pain on your lower back. A kidney stone can generate radiating pain from your back all the way to the front of your torso. There are endless causes of pain. However, some unresolved mental/emotional pain can linger in the body and manifest as physical pain as well.

In my experience, pain—whether it be a slight discomfort or intense suffering—comes from eating low-quality food and holding onto dense, negative emotions without processing them. Most importantly, pain comes from disassociating with those feelings and ultimately losing some aspect of one's self.

I have seen that people who hold onto anger, or harbor resentment from the past, feel physical symptoms of pain. People who eat low-quality junk food and ingest excessive amounts of caffeine feel low energy, experience adrenal fatigue or even exhaustion. Adrenal fatigue occurs when stress triggers cortisol release from the adrenals, which are located right above the kidneys. This can lead to premature aging, slow wound healing, weight gain, muscle breakdown, impaired memory, and a multitude of other health conditions.

I understood that pain was a key component underlying many cases. I also knew that people wanted to avoid pain as much as possible by numbing it with pain-killers, anxiolytics (anxiety medications), alcohol, illegal substances, and food. These are simply other ways of seeking pleasure.

I have encountered patients who came to me in the pharmacy with prescriptions for the same pain medications month after month. Oxycodone, Vicodin, Hydromorphone, Percocet. The prescriptions are the same every month, presented at the same time, like clockwork. As I mentioned, pain can come from a variety of places. Pain is a secondary sign that is sent to an area of trauma or injury. In the case of an actual injury like a torn meniscus or rotator cuff or some other acute condition, pain medication is necessary for temporary relief. When those powerful medications are withdrawn from the body without tapering off appropriately, the person experiences withdrawal symptoms such as nausea, headache, vomiting, and flu-like symptoms.

Opioids bind to the pain receptors and temporarily alleviate pain, but they can also cause tolerance and psychological and/or physical dependency if taken for longer than 6 months. Opiate-dependency becomes such a problem that patients coerce doctors into writing these prescriptions and because pain cannot be measured, doctors have no other choice but to comply and prescribe. In pharmacy, there are so many fears about filling fake prescriptions for Oxycodone because it is the number-one abused prescription medication.

As human beings we want to avoid pain. Who wouldn't? Who would, in their right mind, *seek out* pain?

Prescription-drug overdoses have become rampant in the United States. The National Institute for Drug Abuse reports overdoses recorded for benzodiazepines (Xanax, Valium, Klonopin, etc.), pain-killers, and other prescription drugs. Recent data shows that the highest rise was seen for deaths involving benzodiazepines with a 6-fold increase from 2001 to 2011. This was followed by deaths involving prescription opioid pain-relievers with a 3-fold increase, and deaths involving heroin showing a 2.5-fold increase. Cocaine deaths increased by 22% over the same time period.

I believe all overdoses are preventable with a good plan and the right support system in place. But many of these cases are due to avoidance of emotional pain. Life is too scary or hopeless, and drugs help numb the pain.

Do not misinterpret what I'm saying. Drugs absolutely have their place in treating an illness. If a person cannot function in daily life, temporary use of an antidepressant or anxiolytic (anxiety medication) along with therapy can be extremely useful. Other drugs like antipsychotics may be necessary for someone in an institution. However, so many of those drugs are prescribed in a trial-and-error fashion providing limited relief. The indirect and direct cost to the person taking that medication fans out beyond just the expensive copay with each refill at the pharmacy.

Pharmaceuticals tax the kidneys, liver, and other elimination organs and often produce dramatic side effects, including anything from nausea, headache, tremor, dry mouth, all the way to suicidal thoughts, change in mood, and impulsivity such as gambling and binge eating. Altering brain chemistry has serious effects, especially in developing brains.

In Western society, a person typically seeks medical care when they feel pain or discomfort. We tend to take advantage of our body until it shows signs that something is wrong. Most people won't see a doctor until they show significant symptoms. This is especially true for men. Come on, you know this is true! We will drink excessively, eat like crap, and tax our bodies at work just because we can. Nothing is immediately apparent like a limb falling off or a stroke, but silent damage can occur.

Even when a person does seek medical attention, most of the time they will receive a prescription. There is very little engagement about physical activity or nutrition. And so the silent stresses, poor eating habits, and low activity continue. Most doctors will not even address a condition called pre-diabetes where your blood sugar could be on the borderline of diabetes. Pre-diabetes is defined as having a fasting blood sugar over 100mg/dL. Some doctors do not address this at the point where you can still make significant lifestyle changes. Notice I said *some* doctors not all. I am not attacking the medical community, and I have deep respect for doctors. What I'm saying is that there can be a partnering with health coaches to solve the problem. Integrating health coaches into private practices or clinics can guarantee a continuum of care so each patient has a comprehensive visit.

There is also an expectation to receive a prescription after the visit. We tend to want a "quick fix" especially when pain is concerned. When a patient enters a doctor's office, there is an expectation to receive a prescription at the end of the visit. Say, for instance, you are seeing the doctor for a cough, and you expect to leave with a prescription for an antibiotic. If it is a cold—which is viral, not bacterial, and does not require antibiotics—the doctor will most likely prescribe the antibiotic anyway. A recent study published by the Journal of the American Medication Association showed that 51% of adults over 18 were prescribed an antibiotic for a cough. Doctors inherently want to maintain a strong patient-physician relationship while serving you. They want to make sure they diagnose, treat, and follow up with what is called the "chief complaint," or the main problem you present to them.

The mutual need to maintain a strong relationship between patient and doctor along with comprehensively treating the problem leaves many Western doctors prescribing medication. For example, if someone has an elevated total cholesterol level of 250mg/dL there are guidelines developed by the Adult Treatment Panel III that should be followed. The desirable goal is typically to keep that level below 200mg/dL to prevent stroke and heart attack, and lower cardiovascular risk.

The normal treatment algorithm is to allow the patient to try lifestyle modifications such as diet and exercise for up to 6 weeks, then to try a "statin" or cholesterol-lowering agent if there are no contraindications (reasons why the person cannot take the drug). Often patients leave that consultation with no idea of what a "healthy diet" looks like or "how much exercise" to get. The ambitious patient might Google a healthy diet and implement changes that would lower their cholesterol. More than likely they might return to the office after having their blood rechecked in 6 weeks and be placed on a statin.

Quite honestly, doctors do not have the time to coach patients on healthy eating or exercise, let alone mindfulness techniques such as meditation or how to breathe to ease anxiety and tension. With minimal time to squeeze in a routine physical or office visit, they are pressed for time. Therein lies the crux of the problem in our healthcare system and it is not a new concept. There is so much emphasis on treating disease and minimal efforts to fund preventative efforts such as health coaching.

Our healthcare model is suffering. Attempts to control cost have been implemented within insurance companies. Some pharmacists are involved in teams called a Drug Utilization Reviews (DUR) in which they make an attempt to contain cost through reviewing drug formulary alternatives and helping make informed decisions on how medications are used (called "Medication Therapy Management"). In many cases, the direct and indirect cost to insurance companies rise from frequent hospital visits due to misuse of medication. This is why the pharmacist's role is so important to the healthcare team. Our job is to ensure proper medication use, patient safety, and prevent adverse events that would lead to hospitalization or a doctor's visit.

Addressing preventative care is the optimal solution. Investing in the maintenance of health and preventing illness would save our healthcare system. Many people with chronic diseases such as cancer, diabetes, Multiple Sclerosis, and Rheumatoid Arthritis are susceptible to depression, dysthymia, and anxiety. Learning how to cope with the emotions that may arise upon diagnosis and throughout the illness is pivotal for mental health.

What about when there is pain in the body and no physical trauma that caused it? Why is it there? Where did it come from? You may be saying, *Well, I am not sick. I don't have cancer or diabetes or even depression.* We are all susceptible to pain and illness if we do not process emotions. What we do not process, we store. In the long run, this chronic, low-level stress is what often makes us sick. Traumatic events produce emotions we do not want to feel. Emotions are *energy in motion.* When you bypass processing and feeling, those emotions can make you sick in the future if they remain stagnant in the body. When you do not process emotional traumas, your body responds with pain.

Emotional pain can lie dormant in the chakra system—or the "energy system," which I will explain in more detail later. It's no wonder that stress is the silent killer. According to the Centers for Disease Control, heart disease is the number one cause of death in America. How many of us have had a disappointment or a heartbreak but were convinced we needed to buck up and continue on with our lives? I was always told as a child not to cry in public—to suppress my emotions. I didn't think what I felt was valid or appropriate. Unfortunately I carried that belief into adulthood, which caused me to dissociate from my feelings. Part of unprocessed energy is invested in your cell tissue and is preventing you from being alive, happy, and healthy.

I had avoided feeling for so long that it took physical pain to give me the wake-up call I needed. Someone once told me that when you need to be broken open, God taps lightly on your shoulder. If you do not listen, he shakes you by the shoulder. Finally he hits you over the head with a hammer as if to say, WAKE

UP! This is your awakening to be more than you ever thought possible, to dust yourself off and reveal your inner radiance!

Chapter 3: Craving...oh come on this way please

The clock read 12:58am. Led by the dim lighting above the sink, I maneuvered in a half-dazed state of consciousness into my kitchen. It was my third trip that night to savor yet another piece of bread smothered in peanut butter. Ravenous, I unscrewed the turquoise Skippy lid and layered the creamy, caramel-colored spread onto a chunk of Italian bread. The smooth consistency spilled on my tongue like velvet, bursting into a beautiful symphony of flavor. Another bite. Then another. I barely tasted anything after the first slice. I lost count of how many I'd had and I couldn't control the impulse to consume more. To finally be full. Stuffed and exhausted, I trudged back to bed and collapsed.

The next morning I woke up wanting to die. To hide under the covers forever and stay there wrapped in blankets to cover the heaviness I felt. I trudged to the bathroom avoiding my reflection in the mirror and turned on the sink to brush my teeth and wash my face. All the water in the world couldn't cleanse the guilt and shame I felt. Bloated and tired, I walked to my closet to pick out a loose-fitting shirt and sweatpants to wear to work. I would have to go to the gym at some point. That was for sure. An hour of cardio. Four miles on the treadmill—at least. To undo all of this damage. To fix myself. Another thought popped into my head: maybe later I'll buy some cherry Milk of Magnesia. Not your typical drink of choice on a weekday morning. A bit chalky for my taste. I took note of the previous times I'd chugged a capful of the pink concoction that teetered on what I imagined spackling paste might taste like.

On my drive to work, I thought of David. What would he say if he saw me now? In this ugly, broken-down state? Bags under my eyes, 15 pounds heavier, contemplating driving just a little too far right off the shoulder of the Sunken Meadow parkway and just never quite making it to work?

"Oh, Christina. She was such an outwardly nice, sweet girl. She was going to be a pharmacist. What a shame!" I pictured people lamenting over the obituary in Newsday.

"Sweet my ass," I scoffed, lighting a cigarette, cracking open my car window, and turning up the house music. That was the old Christina. Before shit hit the fan. Before life happened…

I grew up in a typical Italian family. We were taught to work hard, do well in school, and go to college to get an education in a stable, well-paying job. My father was a stoic Italian man. He owned a pharmacy called Winn Drugs that was located on the north shore of Long Island. My father kept all three of his kids busy. Every weekend my siblings and I would have to help him split logs for the fire, rake leaves, or do some new project he had for us. My mother was a sweet, nurturing woman who would literally give you the shirt off her back if you asked for it. She stayed at home with us and drove us around to our activities, cooked, cleaned, and supported us at home.

I was the youngest of three kids. Roy and Lisa were 6 and 8 years my senior, respectively. They fought constantly. Roy would tease Lisa and her friends, and they were always slamming doors.

One night at the dinner table, Roy drizzled Hershey's strawberry syrup into his milk and began instigating Lisa.

"Mom, he's getting the syrup on me!!!" she screamed.

"Roy, sit down. Eat your dinner," my dad yelled and then slapped him hard across the face.

My brother fell silent and obeyed, and my body tensed up. I wanted to vomit or pee my pants—I couldn't decide which. Whenever conflict arose, I immediately got quiet. I didn't want to get hit or sent to my room.

I was always the "sensitive" kid. I cried over everything and I *hated change*. Especially the day I had to leave the comfort of my mother to go to kindergarten. All of us kids lined up single-file outside of the local elementary school, Deauville Gardens. We stood in alphabetical order, where I learned that having a last name at the end of the alphabet would mean I'd have to *wait* for the rest of my time in the public school system.

The Ps were with the Ts so naturally, Tina Pagilaruilo stood in front of me. That day she wore a light green dress with puffy sleeves. Her blonde ringlets bounced in front of my face until she turned around and asked why I was crying.

I didn't want to leave my mother. Why couldn't I just stay home and watch Bob Ross paint those bird-like branches for the green trees and eat my peanut butter sandwich? Why couldn't I be safe and comfortable? I had no choice. I had to go to school.

"Christina it takes three weeks to get adjusted to a new environment. Give it time. You will like your classmates. Enjoy school," my mother would tell me as she lay next to me at night. Of course, she was right as all mothers tend to be, and I would lie in bed at night reciting to my mother each and every person in my class and where they sat in the room. Tina sat to the left behind Eric. Then there was Gina who sat behind Joe when he acted up a lot. I told her how I *hated* lunchtime. The cafeteria was so noisy and I hated sitting with the kids in my class. At times they could be so mean to each other.

As I went on in school I would continue to hate lunch and my sensitivity left me vulnerable for bullying. A group of girls in my fifth grade class began bullying me. I wanted to fit in with them so badly, to be liked and accepted. One day I even ran to the bathroom and felt like I had to vomit but couldn't. I visited the nurse's office several times a week complaining of a stomachache and would lie down on the green couch until my stomach calmed down. I came to terms with the fact that I would have to "deal" with bullies and try to stick up for myself. My parents told me to just suck it up.

Along with school stress, I took on everything my parents challenged me with. I joined the band and played the clarinet, was enrolled in dancing and played basketball or soccer after school— depending on the season. My mother was busy rushing all three of us around to our respective musical and sporting events. My father was busy making sure his drugstore was profitable and could financially provide for us all.

I would cringe to hear my father yell my name from the living room to read history on our worn beige couch. My stomach tightened at the sound of him calling for me. We would sit side-by-side pruning over each paragraph and pausing to reflect on what we had read.

"So what did that paragraph say?" he would ask me.

"I don't know," I'd respond and start to cry.

"Read it again."

"Okay..." I would continue on, burying my anger.

Some nights after he percolated a fire for us, my father would play chess with me, explaining the dance of the pawn and the rook and attempting to lend me the insight of his strategies. We would play Scrabble as a family on Sunday nights. I loved scrambling the words, rearranging the letters on the tile board. Anagrams were my forte. I could look at an anagram in the Sunday paper and unscramble it faster than my father. He was always impressed with how swift I was.

"DIPPED. BRAWN. SPEED. CAUGHT," I'd rattle off after a quick glance at the Sunday paper.

"Damn, you're quick!" he'd say.

Wow. He thinks I'm smart.

I *lived* for that approval. It was like a drug. *Yes, Dad. I am smart.* I did everything I could to get good grades and be a good girl for him.

My father was both an enigma and a wonder to me. I had great respect for him and I also feared him. He always had a project brewing on his mind, whether it was tearing up the rug in the bedroom or tending to the garden or blowing leaves. Even on his days off he would be working outside, pruning the hedges or raking leaves.

Growing up, all I knew was to be busy and to work hard at whatever I did. I would dread the words that spilled from my father's mouth as he asked me to come help him outside. As a young child, I *hated* spending my Sundays working outside.

I distinctly recall one day as a six-year-old hearing my father call my name to come outside.

"Christina! Come help me outside!" he yelled from the back door.

"Mom...I really don't want to..." I whined and began to cry.

"Christina, just go. It won't be long. Maybe an hour," she said.

I wanted to punch a wall, to scream out loud and run away. Yet I knew my personal power was in this man's hands and I had no choice but to wipe the tears off my face, lace up my sneakers, and drag my feet to his newest project.

Every Sunday we would venture out into the shed behind our house. It smelled of sawdust, wood, and old paint. Rows of nails and screws laid in a rusty toolbox, and hammers and screwdrivers lined the walls on wooden racks. I would gaze at the walls, taking in the details of the shed as Dad tinkered around for the right tools.

"Grab me a Phillips head screwdriver," he commanded.

I abided.

"No, you grabbed the flathead. The Phillips has the tapered edge. You see?" he showed me, reaching for a screwdriver with tiny grooves at the end.

We tackled piles of leaves, raking and bagging them one by one. He was a very impatient man. If we ran out of leaf bags and I had to retrieve more, he would yell for me to *run* back to the garage, not walk. And I obeyed, the sound of his booming voice propelling me to run faster. We would chop wood with the log splitter and stack the pieces neatly into a mound.

"Dad, how much longer do we have to stay out here?" I asked one day while we were out tilling about in the yard.

"Don't you ask how long we will be out here. Now we are staying out here longer," he barked back.

I felt so angry, helpless, and scared to speak up to him after that. *I must be bad. I made Dad angry.* Those thoughts seeped into my young mind. It only took one time for me to learn my lesson to never ask that question again. I had to just suck it up for the time being. Keep working. The belief that I was not worthy unless I worked hard sunk deeply into my mind. I came to a silent understanding that my needs and feelings didn't matter. Of course I didn't know the depth of that pain and the conditioned beliefs I would carry into adulthood, so I just kept shoveling and raking and being the good little girl I was supposed to be.

Chapter 4: You're nobody till somebody loves you

As I grew older I began working in my father's drugstore—stocking shelves, sweeping the floor, and tending to the customers at the cash register. My father was a simple man. His idea of a marketing plan was to emboss a neon sign with bold inky pen and post it on a sale rack with cheap Scotch tape. He didn't have a business plan or go to detail his services to doctors' offices. He was perfectly content with the business he bolstered from word-of-mouth. He was, however, extremely resourceful, handy, and always prepared if something broke.

Dad had a certain finesse to ensuring things ran smoothly in the pharmacy, and a personality that I deeply admired. We would often bet that he couldn't make a normally monotone customer laugh and most of the time a corny joke he told would loosen up a smile from the person and he would win the bet.

"Fine, I owe you coffee," I'd scoff in jocularity.

On occasion he would toss empty prescription bottles over his shoulder into our recycling bin as his own goofy way to play solo basketball. He was a kid at heart. I loved every minute of it and as I became more involved in filling prescriptions, the time seemed to pass quicker than a day at a theme park.

At the store I learned the most about people and worked up the courage to talk to them. I would try to ask them about the weather or how their day was going. If they were sick I'd wish them health; if they were distressed I would attempt to comfort them. Behind that counter I felt a connection, an emotional understanding of people's pain and frustrations. It was certainly a humbling experience, as I served customers ranging from the bewildered, hard-at-hearing elderly patients to the jocular residents at the nearby inpatient psychiatric institution. I began to see the various spectrums of behaviors; how people dealt with anger or the death of someone they loved.

And as I grew older and understood what the medications were for, another aspect of these people's lives entered my mind. Conditions such as rheumatoid arthritis, diabetes, hypertension, anemia, schizophrenia, depression, anxiety, and infectious diseases punctured my image of the perfect world. Understanding that people suffered with these diseases opened my eyes to how people dealt with pain.

I wanted to grow into the type of person people knew they could confide in. I wanted to tend to the needs of older people, sick people, young kids, anyone who needed it. I understood how patients needed to feel less anxious when they were starting a new treatment. I developed a deep belief that a pharmacist should assuage their patients' fears and make them feel comfortable. I *needed* to do that. The amount of care I had put into tending to the patients at Winn Drugs led me to believe I was in the right place.

As a 14-year-old cashier, I was in direct contact with people and I thrived hearing their stories, sharing in their pain and pleasure. As I listened to some of them, my eyes would well up with tears, which I quickly wicked away. My sensitive soul had no business crying in public, I reminded myself. I had measured people's ankle size to be fit for a brace, picked out "Confirmation" cards for someone's granddaughter. One day I even put on gloves and gently released the residue from a blister for a customer who had been burned. That physical contact connected me to those patients and gave me an overwhelming feeling of significance. I was hooked.

One day I was working at the register cleaning the countertop after a normal business day. As I was spraying the counter with Windex, I saw one of our regular customers come in flustered and ask to speak to my father. It seemed urgent and I stood back and observed from afar as he listened intently to what she was saying, his eyes focused on hers and his head nodding empathetically as she spoke. He handed her a tissue as tears emerged from her eyes and he embraced her as her body fell listlessly into his arms.

"It's going to be okay. Anything I can do, I'm here for you," I heard him say with compassion.

He lightly touched her arm to reassure her and she thanked him, wiping her tears away.

"Joe. I don't know how to thank you. You have always been there for me and Tony," she said as it dawned on me that her husband had just passed. She took a deep breath and smiled at my father before departing with a look of relief across her face.

And there I was. Standing breathlessly with an unfamiliar expansive feeling in my 14-year-old heart. My chest was exploding with a compelling pull that could only be explained by one word: LOVE. I mean, I loved my parents. I knew what that love felt like.

But this love was different. I had never felt such an intense, all-encompassing emotion in my entire life. I was moved to tears at the sight of such genuine human connection and simultaneously realized that I possessed a yearning to connect with people on a level of magnitude, a depth that would touch them in that same way. I had no idea that capacity even existed, but I knew it was present in me if I was able to recognize it in my father.

Something was whispering to me. That day I heard a tiny voice inside telling me I needed to do that same thing for people for the rest of my life. And from that day on, I couldn't look back. My brain automatically linked pharmacy with love and helping others. My belief was that if I was a pharmacist I could truly make an impact. I became obsessed with making a difference in people's lives — there was no limit to the people I would reach, even on a small scale. I spent my days helping others to achieve that same feeling I felt that day — the heart-centered, loving kindness that can only come from giving to others.

From that day on, I began bringing the Physicians' Desk Reference to Gilgo Beach, memorizing drug names and tiny nuggets of information about them. It brought me joy to know I could someday have the knowledge at my fingertips and deliver it to my patients, translating medical jargon into comprehensible terms. My dad would drive me to work and quiz me on medications, matching generic names to brand names.

"What is the generic of Lipitor?" he asked.

"Atorvastatin," I snapped back, excited I knew the answer.

"Damn, girlie. You're good!" He smiled at me.

"Dad, how do you memorize all of these drugs?" I asked, hungry to know them too.

"You just have to take it one drug at a time, Christina. Just take one drug a day and read about it. Take the package insert off the bottle and devour it."

And that's what I did. I became a garbage-picker, fishing out package inserts from simvastatin bottles, reading about HMG-CoA reductase inhibitors and the side effects that could appear from taking the drug. Any word I didn't know, I looked up. I read about hypertension, cholesterol, diabetes, and other medical conditions all before I even started taking college courses. Nothing would stop me. I was on a mission.

Chapter 5: You're unbelievable, Oh!

Just when I thought I had found *love*, David Bodak walked into my life and everything changed. It was the summer before high school.

It was my 8th grade confirmation when I first saw him and I remember it like it was yesterday. I was sitting in church with my new peach, flower-speckled dress on. Broad shoulders, tall—about 6 foot 4, I estimated. My heart fluttered at the sight of his masculine facial features, strong jaw line and incredible height. He unstitched me. He had a gentleness to him, a sense of calm that I was drawn to like a moth to a light bulb. I walked up to the altar to receive confirmation and barely remember placing the host in my mouth. I just smiled at him as I passed him on my way back to sit down. I knew his sister, Christine, from school. We were in the same grade. In fact, we were really good friends and spent our time together hanging out, walking to Wendy's, or getting Italian ices off of the corner of Merrick Road and Baylawn Avenue in Copiague.

I wanted to meet David and get to know him. I liked his *energy*. It was strong, yet effeminate and pure. One day I was at Christine's house jumping on her trampoline when my mother was supposed to come pick me up. He was washing his mother's car and I was so nervous to go up to him, but I knew if I didn't I would regret it.

"Got some cleaning to do huh?" I said as I touched him lightly. Giddy and breathless, I ran into my mother's car and hoped he would like me. I may have even prayed he would.

Within a couple of weeks, Christine told me that David did in fact like me and wanted to talk to me more. We spent time together and I gave him my phone number. It was easy to be with him. Our energies complemented each other. I was energetic, loud, and loved to be silly. He was mellow, laughed at my corniness, and appreciated me. Cell phones were new back then in 2002 when Nextel had just come out. We texted all the time and I was so excited. I had never "dated" someone before.

He was my first love. Butterflies. Lovey-dovey. Hearts. Love notes. *I <3 U 4EVA.*

We became inseparable. August 5, 2002 would be the day my whole secluded life became worthwhile as I began dating my first boyfriend. I was David Bodak's girlfriend. I had never had a serious relationship before, but I knew being with David made me feel unstoppable, worthy, *alive.*

He helped me through my transition from Middle school to high school. Transitions were never easy and this was no different. Bullies, new teachers, students, and the general unknown scared me beyond belief.

Roy offered me some helpful advice like he always did. "Just keep your eyes on the wall. Don't make eye contact with anyone," he said.

He'd told me stories about vicious high school fights and how he had seen the remnants of girls weaves lining the floor of Copiague High School. Copiague was culturally diverse, enriched with Hispanics, African Americans, Polish — the whole gamete. It didn't faze me — I loved everyone. Gradually my fear subsided and I grew comfortable walking into a classroom shouting out to random people, being absolutely silly and corny. Just like my dad. After a few months, I felt right at home with my new friends and classmates.

I had been on the kickline team in middle school and had made the team in high school. I was still dancing four nights a week at a local studio in Amityville. I loved dancing more than anything because it got out my frustrations and I got to fly across the wooden floor jumping and leaping. It was the one place I knew I could be myself and let loose. I would have kickline practice every day from 3-5 then go to dance from 6-8 or 8-10. I was always busy. School, kickline, dance, homework, David .

I worked at the pharmacy one night a week and on Saturdays. It was a busy pharmacy and we barely had time to eat. When we did, we ate standing up.

"I want to order lunch and eat," I told my sister.

"There's work to do," she said. "But go ahead..." I felt the tense knife of her passive aggressive comment.

"No, it's okay. I'll sticker the order first." An uneasy pang of guilt hit my stomach.

The fast pace got to be too much, even for an energetic 14-year-old. I started to feel extremely tired that October. My dad felt my lymph nodes and said they were "inflamed" and that I should go to the doctor. My blood work confirmed that I had contracted mononucleosis. My body needed rest, but my father had always instilled in us that hard work was the number-one focal point of success. So I kept on dancing and performing in kickline. I kept studying to get good grades in school and working on Saturdays at my father's pharmacy and being a good girl.

One of the immediate effects of mononucleosis that I noticed was a decreased appetite. I only had mono for about 3 weeks but that was all it took for me to lose about 5 pounds and grow accustomed to the attention from looking that much slimmer. My stomach was flat, whereas before it had a little harmless fat. I enjoyed looking skinny and the scale had gone down a whole 5 pounds — I was 123 pounds. From then on I went to kickline without eating a snack like the rest of the girls. I ate a jumbo pretzel with ketchup for lunch and a Lean Cuisine for dinner.

I was genuinely happy. I had a boyfriend who I was in love with, good grades, nice clothes, and a nice body. Everything was so secure and certain. My weight seemed to give me a certain power, a way to control myself. I became addicted to weighing myself at least 3 times a day. I loved being thin. My mom and I would go shopping at Abercrombie and Fitch and I reveled in fact that I was a size 0 or 2. I loved how the frayed shorts would fit my thighs, how slim my arms looked in the mirror. I felt unstoppable, pretty, and lovable. And David loved it, too. He loved *me*.

David and I did *everything* together—from going grocery shopping with his mother to Waldbaum's, to vacations in Montauk, Pennsylvania, and Florida. We took pictures together in Montauk and he made me an album of our journey through the beautiful hills near the lighthouse and the blonde beaches. He lived a 2-minute drive from me in Copiague and we would take turns going over each other's houses for barbecues, walks, bike rides, playing cards, and watching movies. It didn't matter as long as we were together. I fit in with his family. His mom always cooked and had steak on the grill or baked warm blueberry blintzes stuffed with ricotta cheese in the oven. I felt a sense of belonging there. I felt safe.

He was a varsity basketball, lacrosse, and soccer player and I always went to watch his games. Basketball was my favorite to watch. My father and I would go watch David running up and down the court. I would smile and cheer him on, becoming giddy when the announcer called his name.

"Number 33 *David Bodak!!*" His height made for a great guard defender. I was so proud that he was *mine.*

I made sure I knew every player's name, every jersey number, and each player's girlfriend, if they had one.

At the soccer games, I would get eaten alive by bugs, but I loved seeing David dive for the ball. I recall countless Saturdays of watching his home games and even driving to some away games.

When he went to college at St. John's University, I was beyond excited to go see him play lacrosse. On the weekends after work I would drive to Queens and visit him at his apartment. He lived with two other roommates, a basketball player and another lacrosse player. One day I came to the apartment and brought him a box of his favorite granola bars.

"Hey babe. Listen...do you think you could write this paper for me really quick? It's due Monday. I had a busy week with lacrosse and everything," he said as a basketball game buzzed on TV in the background. I paused.

"Um...no..." I said, wondering why he couldn't just do it himself. An inner conflict started festering. My father had always taught us to work hard and this man was clearly lazy.

"Why not?" he asked, surprised.

"Because you should have gotten that done this week. It was due," I said. "Make time for it."

"Haha, she told *you* David," his roommate chimed in, turning from the couch to face us.

"Whatever, fine," David said in a frustrated tone.

I drove home that day and realized that over time David and I had grown apart, not only in physical distance but in our life paths. I was graduating high school and wanted a passionate, ambitious man. David was a Sports Management major and I felt he wasn't serious about getting a steady job.

He was my first, my everything. I learned so much from David —many Polish words, how to drive, and most importantly to have fun without worrying. He took me paintballing for the first time for his senior prom and took the most sacred part of my womanhood. His mother showed me how to make delicious blueberry blintzes and I loved the way she could find any bargain. We even did laundry together in the congested room in his basement. Life with David felt right, orderly, and systematic. Leaving him would throw that all off. It was certain.

After almost 4 years of dating him, I had grown into a different person. I began questioning the direction of my own life as well as what his goals were for the future, whereas he remained stagnant in complacency. I was going to attend St. John's for pharmacy school in the fall of 2006 and I would be faced with another transition— from high school to college. Except this time I was doing it without him. I had to leave. I had to step into the unknown for the first time in my life and experience *life*.

Chapter 6: All I wanna say is that they don't really care about us

Leaving David wasn't as easy as I thought it would be. I was like a weak fawn learning how to walk again.

Everything reminded me of him—smells, places we used to eat, certain foods, even specific phrases replayed in my mind like it was straight out of a movie, a caricature of our lives together. Any time I would visit the Roosevelt Field Mall, I would recall all of those times we walked into American Eagle, Hollister, or Abercrombie and Fitch. And each time I would smell his Sean Paul cologne lingering on the cuff of someone else's shirt I felt as if I were riding a bicycle with no hands—out of control and groundless. Inevitably I would cry, reliving memories from our past. I cried every single day.

The reel of memories would start late at night. My mind would make up scenarios, picturing him and his roommates watching sports and relaxing to the din of sportscasters' melodies catching up on past basketball games and picking football drafts. I could never relate to these events, but I remember loving the arcane language of plays and players' names that my father and David spoke about. That dialogue never made sense, but I loved listening as I got ready for our dates while David and my dad conversed in the living room. I loved his tall stature and how he could carry me anywhere—the way he took a bite out of a chicken parm hero and held his fork with his sausage-like fingers. But mostly I missed how he seemed to have unconditional love for me.

That had all slipped away much like my innocence as I prepared for college at St. John's in 2006. Who was I if I wasn't David Bodak's girlfriend? If I wasn't a dancer or a perfect student? How was I going to handle this? David was going to the same college as me, I had to live with 8 new people, move away from home, take on a completely new course-load, and try to have a social life to squeeze the most out of what is supposed to be "the best years of your life." Damn, that was a lot of pressure.

But I was so excited at the same time—I had waited four years to get to this place. I couldn't wait to get to college and soak up what I'd yearned to understand for years. I would learn about alpha blockers, calcium channel blockers, thiazide diuretics, HMG-CoA reductase inhibitors. How did a pharmacist know if two drugs interacted? That would be the deliciously fun part, and I would savor every bit.

The first wisps of responsibility, pressure, and fear snaked its way into my life that August. No one was there to protect me as I grappled with anxiety and other emotions I wasn't prepared to handle. An overpowering mixture of feelings plagued me—regret, disappointment, loneliness, guilt, rejection, hopelessness. I would drive past David's house at night, park at the foot of the hill of Pleasantview Court, and reminisce of the times we'd had together. I felt completely empty, although I didn't want to believe it or even acknowledge it. So I did what a normal teenager would do—keep busy, go out, and party.

When I got to college the food they offered in the dining hall consisted of unlimited amounts of pancakes, waffles, fries, chicken nuggets, and a fully stocked ice cream and dessert bar. There were so many opportunities to visit the dining hall with study groups and friends, and come home from the bar late at night to eat. With endless papers and lab reports due, even in my first year of pharmacy school, I found myself constantly reaching for comfort food. In fact, I got up every night to eat cereal, cookies, and peanut butter. This was such an odd behavior and caused me daily emotional pain and anguish because I had been trim my entire life. I had been "perfect" and this completely dissembled me. I couldn't understand why this night eating syndrome had started.

I buried my heart in love and food. I wanted so badly to meet someone else to fill the void, to have someone love me like David did. Roy invited me out with his friends to nightclubs where they knew people so I could get in even though I was only 18. Secretly I was hoping for another opportunity to find someone to love me.

My first club was Club One in Astoria. I went with my brother and his girlfriend at the time. The loud techno music pumped out through the door as people were let in. The flashing colorful lights coming from inside of the club excited me as I waited impatiently in the summer humidity. I wore a conservative white tank top and short jean shorts. I just wanted to dance and let loose. The tough-looking bald bouncer scanned my fake ID, ignoring the picture of my once-thin young face from years prior. He stamped my hand and the door was opened for me, a cool rush of air painting my skin fading behind loud house beats.

I *loved* loud house music! My brother had always driven me in his blue Honda Accord late at night with the windows down blasting it. I got lost in the wordless trance as we sped down Deer Park Avenue. He would put the air conditioning on, roll the windows down, and blare the music. I was out of control inside. The erratic pulses and waves gave me strength. It made me think there was more out there than just the dull parameters I had merely brushed upon in my immature life.

The party scene was enticing and I constantly thrived on going out and dancing. It got my crazy, out-of-control feelings out. After a night of dancing and failure to meet anyone who truly understood me, the disappointment and loneliness would be compounded, more out of control because I was miserably alone. Little did I know the psychology of the average teenage guy. I met guys and a lot of them wanted to kiss and grab me. They wanted to dance and grind on me and it was all fun in the moment. But there was no solace to be found at nightclubs. I was completely alone in a room full of people.

One night after a club, about a week before my 18th birthday, I stumbled into my house tipsy and hungry. You know that drunken hunger pang that needs to be filled even though you shouldn't be compounding heavy food with alcohol at wee hours of the morning? It was a humid June night and the fireflies always come out around that time, with honeysuckle plants emerging in the southwest corner of my house. I went into the kitchen cabinets and poured myself some Kashi GoLean cereal and passed out in my bed. I woke up an hour later and was still hungry. I meandered into the kitchen and poured myself another bowl of cereal. The cold milk hit my lips and the crunchy texture satiated my hunger. Ah...sweet, cold, hearty. I was full. I passed out again and woke up feeling groggy the next day. The sugar crash combined with lack of sleep left me fatigued and cranky.

The next night I woke up with the same craving. I needed to eat; I was starving. My body was primed to get up an hour after I went to sleep from that night on. The next time I went for bread and peanut butter. Night after night, I would wake up and eat. Sometimes multiple times a night. It was as simple as that—the pattern was formed after about a week. I was half awake when I ate it. The creamy, rich, full-bodied texture of peanut butter tasted sinful to me. Pretty soon that big Skippy jar with the turquoise top became my biggest enemy. It was like I couldn't control myself, or my choice to eat. And it was all a big secret.

Since I had been anorexic a few years before, I felt like a huge failure. During the day I would have Diet Cokes and eat salads, avoiding carbohydrates so I wouldn't gain more weight. I exercised as much as possible, beating up my body every day just to maintain this image that I was still "normal." After all, I was *trying* to be normal, trying to convince *myself* I wasn't completely and utterly *fucked up.* All day these judgmental thoughts entered my mind. *Why are you doing this? What's wrong with you? You used to be so thin. Who will love you now that you're gaining weight?* Those thoughts only deepened the habit. I began eating more.

My entire family was slim and healthy. My sister had a beautiful body: perfect, robust chest, and small waist. I felt like an outcast on so many levels, but I knew my brother had the same habit since he was 7 years old.

One day I was at the beach and my brother said to me, "Wow, looks like you put on a couple of pounds, Christina."

"Shut up, you asshole. You do the same thing," I retorted, recalling countless nights of seeing my brother rummage through the kitchen cabinets in the middle of the night.

Maybe it was genetic? Why was this eating disorder coming out now? I tried to rationalize it, analyze it, take it apart and bury it all at once. My thoughts just dug it deeper.

I got so fed up with the habit that I decided to begin researching it. Maybe I wasn't the only one doing this. My brother had exhibited this behavior as well as my aunt and grandfather — maybe other people did it, too. Apparently, it had a title, an actual diagnosis in the Diagnostic and Statistical Manual of Mental Disorders (DSM) IV: Night Eating Syndrome. Patients who had taken the prescription sleeping aid, Ambien, and had dieted had exhibited the same behavior. Since Ambien shuts off the conscious part of the brain, the unconscious parts take over while the person is sleeping. So if the person really wants chocolate cake and the conscious part is being subdued by the drug, they got up to eat. There were reports of people eating entire chocolate cakes or plates of lasagna. I didn't gorge myself on an entire cake, but I knew my behavior wasn't normal.

I read about one patient on Ambien who said, "I would wake up in the morning and there would be candy wrappers all around the bed. There would be crumbs in the bed. There would be all kinds of evidence that someone had been eating in the bed. But I had absolutely no recollection of it."

I read on….

Night Eating Syndrome is classified as a sleep disorder. The classic symptoms include morning anorexia, with at least 50% of calories consumed after dinner. Secondary effects include weight gain, disrupted sleep, agitation, depression, fatigue throughout the day, and emotional instability. The disorder has a genetic component and is most common in young women, effecting about 2% of the population. In my case, my maternal grandfather, my aunt on my mother's side and my brother all had periods of symptomatic NES. A stressful event compounded with a family history could cause Night Eating Syndrome. As many as 25% of bariatric surgery patients met the criteria for NES. My mind was blown.

People who have NES are reported to have an altered Hypothalamic-pituitary-adrenal (HPA-axis), which regulates stress hormones. Cortisol, a hormone produced by the adrenal glands which are located on top of the kidneys, are activated when a person is under stress. Excessive stress and increased levels of cortisol lead to weight gain, fat deposits especially in the gut and midsection, lowered immunity, suppressed thyroid function, and cognitive performance. Researchers have hypothesized that NES may result from experiences of stress that manifest into cravings for certain foods. Increased levels of stress can result from occupational or personal distress, exacerbating the condition and increasing anxiety at night. NES sufferers lack melatonin, the hormone released at night to induce sleep, as well as serotonin, the neurotransmitter that regulates mood and appetite.

I stopped reading. All of these things were true. I ate 50% of my calories after bedtime, mostly carbohydrates and sugar. I pinched the fat around my stomach and cringed, reminiscing of the flat stomach I had but 6 months prior when everything was *normal*.

I was 18 and way too scared to talk to anyone about what I was doing. I was getting up at night and bingeing on peanut butter and pretzels, pizza, whatever had carbohydrates and tasted good. How embarrassing! It was my medicine, my therapy. It felt good to eat and feel full before going back to sleep. In fact, I couldn't go back to sleep without eating.

I avoided social situations with food and was scared to eat around people, even my family. The level of shame was too intense.

"Christina, come out to dinner with us. We're going to Ciao Baby," my mom would say.

"Nah, not hungry," I retorted.

"Just come! Stop moping around," my dad said.

"No, you guys go. I'm tired," I would respond and head into my bedroom, relishing the solitude. I had no time to think about this eating disorder. I was too occupied with college and starting the rest of my life, and goddamn it, I was going to revel in it.

Chapter 7: Whoa, we're halfway there, whoa, livin' on a prayer

"Guys, are you ready yet?!" I yelled from my dorm room.

"Christina…it's 8:30. We aren't leaving 'til 10," Tonya said, still in her pajama pants.

"Oh. Yeah." I swiveled around to waste another hour and a half. I opened up my Biology book and sat on the top bunk, my boots dangling off the side of the bed. I got lost in the chambers of the heart, how each valve opened and closed in perfect harmony. How did the body work in such a marvelous systematic way? Effortlessly…beating in sync….

"Christina! Get up!!" Tonya screamed.

My eyes shot open. The biology book lay open over my chest, to the page explaining the function of the cord-like tendons of the chordae tendinae.

"We leaving?" I asked in a groggy voice.

"Yeah, get your ass up. I'm ready to partayyyyy!!!"

Anthony from down the hall appeared in the doorway. "Tarantula! Come on down. We're headed to Last Call," he said.

We strutted past the guards near Gate 6, ready for our badass excursion of under-aged drinking. The size of Last Call felt more like someone's shoe closet than a college bar, but we squeezed in and managed to reach over people to order our drinks.

"Two Long Island iced teas," I barked at the bartender.

"Quick and dirty," I said, turning around and handing Tonya her drink.

"Where are the hot guys around here, man? Need to go to Harvard or Villanova to get some guys with *substance*," Tonya insisted.

"Haha. You're funny. I just want a tall guy. Someone to have fun with," I said, sipping my drink.

Just as those words left my lips, Paul Roecker walked through the door, high-fiving one of his fraternity brothers.

"Oh my God. There's Paul!" I whispered to Tonya. "Talk about someone I'd want to have fun with..." My eyes fixated on his brown hair sprouting out of the sides of his dark blue Yankee hat. He lived in DaSilva hall, the dorm adjacent to mine, and he was in my Biology class.

Tonya shouted over the music. "Oh, you know you love those intellectual types. He's in the PA program, right?"

"Yeah. Don't be so loud, T. I need another drink. You done with your LI Tea yet?" I pressed, my eyes following Paul as he edged closer to the bar, making his rounds to say hi to everyone.

"Damn, girl. I knew you were from Long Island, but I didn't know you could chug one like a fish!" she exclaimed.

"Come on, let's go get another one." I grabbed her hand and nudged past the crowd of college freshmen to get to the bar.

"Buckets! How the hell are ya?!" I heard a familiar voice from behind me shout.

"Oh, hey Paul!" I turned around and almost spilled my fresh Long Island Iced Tea on his plaid shirt.

I reflected on the nickname Buckets he had given me after we joked that David's nickname had been Mr. Buckets and was also the name of the toy, Mister Buckets. *Mister Buckets, put the balls in my mouth.*

"I'm great. A little bit drunk. But feeling good." I smiled up at him. I loved being able to look up at a tall guy. It made him seem more masculine. It made me feel safer.

"You look gorgeous tonight," he said.

"Thank you." I batted my eyelashes and moved in closer to him, taking in the intoxicating smell of beer on his breath.

"Did you lose weight?!" he asked.

"Are you kidding? Ugh, I used to be a lot thinner. My sister is the thin one in the family!" I said loudly and then quieted my voice abruptly, realizing how much my voice projected even in the noisy bar.

"Nah. You are a hottie, Tarantola." He winked. "Listen, I'm gonna go catch up with a few friends and play a round of pool. See you in a bit?"

My heart sank. "Yeah, totally. Sure. See you later." I turned around and gulped down a huge sip. *Fuckin' idiot. Why did you say that? Probably turned him off.*

I looked around as 20-somethings, my peers, laughed and shared pitchers of beer with their friends. Across the room, sorority girls posed in a group picture on the pool table. One girl grabbed a pool stick, posed, and made a peace sign. "Upload this to Facebook!" she said after her friend took the picture.

Some girl right in front of me was making out with a guy, tongue down his throat as they nestled in the corner of the wooden table. They were in a full-on make-out session. They held my attention until I felt stomping on the table next to me. I looked up and saw girls dancing and belting out the lyrics to "Livin' on a Prayer" by Bon Jovi. The entire bar sang in unison and I felt the vibration of the bass throughout my whole body.

"Whooah, we're halfway there
Whoaaah, livin' on a prayer
Take my hand and we'll make it – I swear
Whoa, livin' on a prayer"

I joined in and sang at the top of my lungs, grabbed Tonya's hand and thanked God I was alive and in this crowded, sweaty bar with my quirky, sassy, incredibly up-for-anything best friend. This was *life*. And I was living it.

The next day I woke up with a pounding headache and cotton mouth. *Too many Long Island iced teas. How did I even get home?*

I looked down at my clothes and saw that I had been conscious enough to change into my blue Copiague High School t-shirt but forgot to put on any pants. Fiber One cereal lie scattered on my turquoise sheets intermingled with raisins. As I got up to reach for my water, raisins fell to the ground.

Fuck. Did I wake up Juleen?

Juleen was my roommate who slept on the bottom bunk. She was known for bringing home guys and also bringing home the distinct smell of lubricant and lust with her boyfriend of the week.

I quickly rushed down the ladder of my bunk bed to retrieve the evidence of the raisins. Sweeping the cereal off the bed, I sighed and turned to see the time. It was only 7:00am.

I felt my bloated stomach and looked around the room in the darkness. The slits of light from the blinds reflected on my two roommates as they lay silently dreaming away. I envied their restful sleep and longed for the day that I could have a normal night's sleep, if that even existed. I felt nauseated and worthless after the alcohol, carbohydrates, and lack of sleep. I put on stretchy black yoga pants and yanked on my beige Ugg boots.

Ten minutes later I arrived at the Rite Aid off of Parsons Avenue and Union Turnpike. Peering down the vitamin aisle, I looked to see who was around. An old woman perusing the Centrum Senior vitamins. *What would she care if an 18-year-old was buying diet pills?* Passing the Omega 3s, B-complex and multivitamins, I came across the diet pills and quickly scanned a box for something that would work quickly. A generic weight-loss supplement, 60 count. *That'll do.*

I buzzed over to the stomach relief aisle and plucked a box of chocolate Ex-Lax off the shelf along with a bottle of cherry Milk of Magnesia. Rushing to the register, I felt a surge of urgency and guilt. *At least no one knew me here.* I drove near 179th street and put the car in park. I ripped the plastic off the top of the bottle with my teeth and poured the liquid Milk of Magnesia into the cup. *Take a swig like a champ. Ugh, fucking horrible. Tastes like shit.* My stomach rumbled and I took a hard swallow as a pang of remorse overwhelmed me.

Chapter 8: This is ourselves…under pressure

"Christina, why are you taking Ex-Lax?" my mother asked me, quizzically. "I saw it in your desk drawer," she answered my question before I could ask it.

"Why are you going through my desk drawer?" Already, my anger was mounting.

"What's wrong? Tell me. Is it the night eating?" she asked gently, attempting to pull the answer from me. She had caught me binge eating after I had been rummaging through a bag of pretzels a week prior.

"I'm fine, Mom."

"Are you sure you don't want to go see someone? Remember Adrienne from The Spoon? We saw her and she did the psychic reading on us?"

"Um, yeah. What does that have to do with therapy? She's a psychic, not a therapist," I retorted, guarding my ego.

"She does private counseling, too. I spoke to her earlier today…" I could tell my mom was walking on eggshells, anticipating my anger.

"What?! Mom. I'm fine. Seriously. Why did you call her?"

"You haven't been happy, Christina. Now I find these pills? I think it would be a good idea to go. At least once. Just think about it, okay?"

"Yeah, I'm gonna go for a run," I said, lacing up my sneakers and grabbing my head phones.

Fuck—am I really that bad? No one else seems to notice. Dad hasn't said anything about my performance at work. I'm still pretty functional. Nah, I don't need a shrink. What could this person tell me that I don't already know?

Turning up the house music on my phone, I drowned out the thoughts and kept running.

Throughout school, I *survived*. I was determined and had the goal in mind to serve my patients and nothing would get in the way of that. It wasn't easy considering I was waking up countless times a night and eating carbohydrates, waking up groggy and restless.

But I was a fake at school. A complete phony. I felt like I had two faces hiding behind a façade.

"Hi Michelle! How was your weekend?!" I'd find my seat in the front row next to the other overachievers.

I'd just finished off a Parliament light and a large coffee from 7-11. I hated myself. I was grossly aware of how tight my pants were fitting—I had gained at least 20 pounds.

Why did you eat those chips last night?

Class would start. I sat in the front row every single class, with my eyes peeled, ears open, devouring the material. We learned about pathology, how the disease process manifests in the body. We dissected rats in anatomy lab and named each tissue and organ in the body. In Drugs and Disease we layered what the drug structure looked like with how it bound to each tissue in the body and how it was metabolized and excreted. We were required to know the mechanism of action and exactly how the drug would bind to the receptor site. The details required for that class alone was grueling; everyone dreaded 4th-year Drugs and Disease classes. And that was only one course. We had 18 credit semesters, which translated to 21 hours with our lab days.

I stayed focused. I knew what I wanted and I would get it. Sick or not. During class, my mind would start up...

Okay, so after this I'll go to the gym. Run 5 miles to burn off those chips. That'll be good. Fuck, I'm tired today. Then I'll study for Organic Chemistry. Exam Friday. I'm hungry again – it's 11am but I ate too much last night. I don't deserve to eat again. Maybe I'll eat a salad when I get home later.

"What are you doing today after class? Studying for the midterm?" Michelle asked, breaking me from my thoughts.

"Yea. Then going to the gym for a bit. Maybe writing after that," I said.

"Christina, you are *so* good with time management! How can you go to the gym, study, *and* have a social life?"

"Ah, I guess I just get things done quickly."

The real answer? *Classical conditioning. Determined Type A. Demanding father.*

I got things done for sure. As or Bs in every class, gym 6 times a week, out at the bar every Wednesday and Friday night. It was so much easier to avoid any thoughts of David that way. My life was all shiny and held together on the outside for a while, but then I started to fall apart.

Chapter 9: You make me sick, I want you and I'm hatin' it...

The stomach pains came in droves. Intense bouts of stomach pain right above my navel. It was so unbearable I couldn't get up in the morning. Plus I was extremely tired, so I had no motivation to move. I pushed myself to go to school, work, and maintain my life as best as I could. But it was so debilitating that I had to go to my doctor to see what was wrong with me.

I was 18 when I walked into Dr. Desposito's office. I sat upright perched on the exam table, shifting my weight uncomfortably and feeling the white sanitary paper rustle beneath me. He examined my tongue, my ear canals, palpated my stomach, and asked where it hurt.

"All over, not really anywhere specific..." I said, my voice trailing off, eyes wandering to the crevices of the old office ceiling.

"Okay, you can sit up, Christine." He called me by the wrong name as most do. My ultimate *pet peeve.*

"Sometimes people get stomach pain from things that cause stress. It seems you may be depressed," he explained.

The words coated my brain like a thick layer of goo. D-E-P-R-E-S-S-E-D.... It seemed to repeat slowly. Immediately I started crying. The mental chatter returned—*I'm 18, why am I depressed? How do I take this away?*

"I can prescribe you something that will help you deal with this," he offered with good intent.

"NO. I don't want it," I said abruptly. You would think that a future pharmacist would embrace medications. After all, don't you practice what you preach? In reality, most pharmacists do not take medications because we know so much about how they affect the body. I would find any other way to correct my chemical imbalance. It was my mission and nothing would stop me.

As the old adage goes, "Whatever you resist, persists." Inevitably, food and clubs didn't resolve my pain so I finally agreed to go see Adrienne DeSalvo. My mother and I had met this woman at a local coffee shop a few months prior for a psychic reading. Apparently she also offered counseling for people in grief. I recalled the intense emotion that resulted at the restaurant on Wellwood Avenue the night I met Adrienne. How she called upon my grandfather and past relatives who had passed away years ago only to find specific details of my life that no one else could have known. I remembered Adrienne's calmness, her tranquil aura. After months of intense grief and desperate denial and avoidance, I decided to help myself.

It was time for therapy. The dreaded 'talk therapy' for the labeled weak and wounded. I couldn't understand why I was getting up at night eating junk food. I couldn't grasp why I felt like sleeping all day, and why my stomach was constantly hurting. Mostly, I couldn't grasp why I hadn't felt happy in months. I wanted answers, and I was willing to have my mother drive me to this woman's house to find them.

The initial visit to the basement apartment in Adrienne's house was one of the toughest things I'd ever brought myself to do. It took actual effort to not run away as I approached the door that December day after my mother dropped me off. My inner child was kicking and screaming.

"Good luck, honey! Don't cry too much. Or make a complete ass of yourself!" I pictured my mother shouting as she booted me out of the car. My mother would never say such a thing. She was a kindhearted woman who did absolutely anything anyone asked of her.

At that time I knew I needed help and perhaps this woman could do whatever it was therapists were meant to do. I wasn't sure of the outcome, but there was a good chance that the costly session had to bring some relief. So much fear flooded my body as I knocked on the door and a tiny 4 foot 11 older woman appeared with a smile. She invited me inside and quickly apologized for the messy apartment.

I'm not worried about how your apartment looks, love, I'm an emotional mess.

Upon our start of the session, she explained her purpose to help me gain insight into my emotions, which are ultimately connected to thoughts and behaviors. After she offered me a glass of water, I immediately started crying and requested a box of tissues. I had a difficult time finding the words to implicate my feelings as she questioned where all of my anxiety stemmed from. What were the problems I'd encountered in my past? What relationships had I experienced?

In dribs and drabs, and between sniffles and a quivering voice, I told her the story of David.

"Honey, how do you feel?" she asked when I was finished.

How do I feel? Well, no one has ever asked me that question. What are feelings? I know these terms, but I have never attached meaning to them. All I felt was tired, so I went with that.

"I'm tired. That's all I know. No one has ever talked to me about feelings." I blew my nose into a soggy tissue.

"Okay. Well let's start here," she said, pulling out a piece of paper with pictures of dozens of faces with expressions on them — each face had a feeling word beneath it. Angry. Sad. Frustrated. Tired. Lonely. Guilty.

I felt like I was in KINDERGARTEN. But I remained open.

"Most people don't assess their feelings," she explained. "They perform daily activities without realizing what they feel and how to release those emotions in a healthy way."

Was this the crux of therapy? To acknowledge, feel, and then release feelings? *I can do that,* I resolved.

Adrienne DeSalvo — "salvo" meaning safe — became my "safe space." One of the first things I learned from her was that **"It all**

goes back to the feelings." I had to learn to process my feelings in order to heal.

As challenging as it was, the next week I returned to her cozy apartment filled with giraffe statues, owl posters, and heart-shaped rocks.

Something about this woman made me feel comfortable. She was a free spirit and had maternal tendencies. Within the next few sessions, I grew to trust and love her as a mentor and friend. Each week she would listen and comment on the feelings I may have overlooked, and question me on what I was thinking or feeling when certain events occurred. We pieced together possible sources of anxiety that would contribute to night eating, and differentiated between physical and emotional hunger. I was an *emotional eater*. I occasionally asked her about her life and she drew upon her own experiences to teach me of her divine ways. I soon learned Adrienne was kind, forgiving, inspired, motivated, spiritual, grateful, loving, and compassionate. I admired her deeply.

As our relationship grew and our sessions progressed, Adrienne introduced me to a multitude of tools to cope with my feelings. We maneuvered through conversations about the ego and how many people in society run their lives unconscious of their own thoughts and feelings, thus creating stress and worry for others. She introduced me to Eckart Tolle's book *The Power of Now*, Melody Beattie's *The Language of Letting Go*, and *In the Meantime* by Ylana Vanzant. We spoke about meditation, prayer, and yoga, practices completely unfamiliar to me then. Her calm disposition and strong belief that these tools would work for me led me to become voracious to understand more about spirituality, living in the present, dealing with emotions, and meditating.

I began opening up to my mother about my eating disorder and we had countless talks over coffee in our glass sunroom. Often my mother and I would take a drive down to the Lindenhurst docks and just stare out at the darkness illuminated by the stars. We would revel in the passage of time, the current season or the boats encased in shrink-wrap tided over for the winter. On numerous occasions I would pour my heart out to her about my inner battle or any relationship problems I was having, and she would listen patiently, offering advice as best as she could. The weight of my problems seemed lighter after each of our drives to the docks.

Adrienne and I talked so much about feelings, and I had a ton of them. She recommended I keep a journal to get to know myself and "get those feelings out on paper" to disperse some of the anxiety. I began to journal almost every day, words pouring out of me onto blank sheets of paper, onto Microsoft Word documents, onto sticky notes—any loose piece of paper I could find. I became enamored with the way words could calibrate emotion. A simple word choice could ignite a shiver up your spine, bring a tear to your eye, or cause you to shudder in fear.

I wanted to share my new insights with everyone, to inspire others who were struggling with similar challenges. So I began writing Facebook notes. I wrote about all of the things college kids struggled with such as alcohol, emotions, stress, and especially troubles of the heart. It started out as a general desire to share my thoughts, and turned into something completely unexpected. People started complimenting my work, saying I was insightful and perceptive. Motivated and enthralled, I began writing weekly on Facebook.

Adrienne always told me, "It takes courage to express yourself and share with people what you think and feel." I knew I was being vulnerable, but I loved touching people and relating to them, allowing my classmates to know they weren't alone in their struggles throughout college. For the next year and a half, I maintained my note-writing and ended up with more than 100 notes. I knew I wanted to write a book, but I couldn't figure out what my story would be about. I knew I wanted to inspire people, to allow people to read about my experiences and decide for themselves which path to take.

I began connecting with nature and started writing in Long Beach. My mood lifted. I had always loved the water as a child. My family and I had gone to Gilgo Beach for years, but my mother and I discovered it after my uncle had completed a fundraiser for the Polarbear Club, where in the dead of winter everyone gets into their bathing suits and dives into the ice-cold water. After just one visit, I was hooked.

I would go to the beach to run on the boardwalk or to sit and write as people buzzed around me. I couldn't get enough of the serene water or the confluence of people running, playing with their children, or sunning their tan bodies. I wrote countless journal entries about Long Beach, each one pouring out of me as I drew inspiration from peering out into the ocean water. The feel of the boardwalk under my bare feet or the colorful display of the warm reds and oranges of the Long Island sunset could instantly quell my fears about life.

Being alone felt safe. I consulted solace near the Atlantic Ocean with my pen and leather-bound journal in hand. It allowed me to create space in the incessant stream of thoughts that ran through my mind every other second of the day. I viewed life with such vibrancy, as if the fog had been lifted from my field of vision. The smell of a barbecue grill or the feeling of the cool breeze grazing my skin after a run in Long Beach would put a smile on my face. The simplicity of a butterfly gently floating by took me into another dimension.

Life came alive, and nothing mattered but being in the present. I was genuinely happy in those moments. I held them so closely to my heart and was brought to tears by the amount of beauty I had missed out on for so many years.

On the days I ran in Long Beach, I felt free, expanded, boundless, and connected. To what? To whom? To myself. To nature and every being on the planet. I felt it at the deepest part of my being, but I couldn't rationalize it. I felt it in my own beating heart. Beyond the physical plane, I knew there was some being watching over me, providing for me and guiding me. It was faith. It was against everything I had ever been taught or fed growing up. Yet there was a *knowing* deep inside.

My father did not believe in God or anything that couldn't be explained scientifically. If he put work into something, he wanted to see the fruits of his labor. Faith and trust were too whimsical to grasp and were not in his vernacular. But it was in those silent moments at Long Beach as I listened to the undulating waves near the shore that I began believing in something more powerful, universally encompassing, and eternal. It was there that I began to cultivate faith in God.

Chapter 10: Stay or leave, I want you not to go but you should...

I was still hooked on my two main drugs—food and love. I had added a third, cigarettes. It kept my weight down and blunted my appetite. I was up to running 5 miles a day.

I craved connection and love and I was absolutely obsessed with Paul Roecker from my chemistry class. We had hooked up a year prior on Halloween even though he had a girlfriend at the time. He left abruptly the next morning. We were both drunk and his girlfriend went to school upstate somewhere, so I rationalized that it didn't really count. It stung when she came to visit him a month later and I saw them out at Last Call. I didn't care. The deep desire for love left me like a drug addict and I wanted him. We still spoke occasionally and decided to meet up.

"So we are meeting around 10:30, right? Rockville Center," I texted him.

I checked my phone every minute after.

"Yeah," he wrote back an hour later.

"Okay, see you then!" I replied right away.

"Let's go to RJ Daniels first. I need to get a couple drinks in me before I see him," I told my friend Jackie. I needed a wing-woman to deal with this.

"Okay, that sounds good. They have two-fers on Fridays!"

It was 10:00 and the inside portion of the bar was already packed. Everyone was too cold to stay outside despite the plastic overhang covering that part of the bar.

"Yeah, can I have two orders of vodka seltzer with lime?" I said to the tall, dark, and handsome bartender.

"Sure," he said, grabbing a bottle of Svedka and effortlessly squirting bubbly club soda into a glass. He never smiled at me, although I wished he would have. I tried to make eye contact with him, but he didn't seem interested.

I couldn't wait to see Paul—he was quirky, creative, and intelligent. His somewhat long black hair turned me on, and he exuded confidence. I wanted him to want me. He rarely gave me the time of day...up until now.

I remembered how he made me feel as he kissed me hard that Halloween night after we got back to my apartment. Busting through the front door of my apartment, he had unzipped my coat the rest of the way as I giggled in drunken bliss. My roommate at the time, Ann Marie, was watching TV in her room with the door slightly open. I ignored her presence and grabbed at his belt as we made our way to my room and slammed the door shut. He unhooked my bra with one hand, maneuvering his hands all over my chest, my stomach.

"Ugh, you have a *fucking* amazing body, Christina," he'd said, lustfully.

My mind snapped back into focus as I saw him walk through the door, red and black plaid shirt, dark blue jeans, and hair messy. I waited for him to scan the crowd for me.

"Tina! How are yaaaaa?" He smiled.

"Great. Who'd you come with?"

"A couple of friends from Lynbrook. How about you?" he asked.

"My friend Jackie." I pointed to my bubbly blonde friend.

"You know what...I have to go to the bathroom," he said.

"I do too. Want walk there together?" I asked.

"Ugh...sure." His tone sounded uncertain.

We headed for separate bathrooms and I told Jackie I'd be back in a minute. I primped my curly hair and applied my clear lip gloss. Fixing my denim skirt and pulling up my black stockings, I decided I looked pretty damn sexy. I headed outside and looked around for Paul. Nowhere to be found...

"Where did you go?" I texted him.

No answer. Ten minutes went by. Then twenty. I needed another drink. And a cigarette. This was not happening.

I dialed his number, blowing a puff of smoke into the cold winter breeze.

"Hello," he answered abruptly.

"Hey...ummm where did you go?"

"My friend threw up," he said matter-of-factly. "I had to take him back to Lynbrook."

"Are you coming back?" I asked.

"I might."

"I'll wait. How long will you be?" I asked hopefully.

"Probably won't come back. I'm too drunk," he said.

"That's such *bullshit!* Are you fucking kidding me? You had just gotten to the bar. You weren't drunk at all."

"Whoa. I drank when I got back here, Christina," he said defensively.

"Yo, you always do this shit. You say you're coming through and you play these fuckin' games. Or I see you once and then not again for six months. See you again in six months when you decide to text me."

"I'm not your boyfriend," he yelled. "Don't talk to me like that."

I hung up. The tears came. I was drunk. I was emotional. I needed to leave. I needed to stop chasing people who couldn't love me.

Jackie drove me home and I cried the entire way. *Why can't I get over this person? Why do I seek love from people who won't give it to me?*

"Jackie, can I sleep at your house tonight? I don't want to be alone tonight." I felt like a little kid asking to sleep in the bed with their parents.

"Sure, Christina. Hey, I love you. Don't be upset. He doesn't deserve you! You'll find someone else," she said, trying to comfort me.

"Yeah…probably…." We got to her house and I was miserable. I was so glad I didn't have to sleep alone again. I was so happy I wouldn't wake up once, twice, three times to numb my feelings with food and avoid feeling the pain of rejection. Mostly I was happy I wouldn't have to betray myself over and over again.

Chapter 11: Stop playin' with my mind

After that night, I knew I needed to pick myself up and move forward to improve my life. I was a goddamn mess. I remembered my father had been hypnotized for weight loss and I wondered if a hypnotist could help with night eating. I searched online for a hypnotist in the city. Maybe this would work for me.

Dialing the number on the website, I prayed this man could help me.

"Hello, Doug Oconnor speaking," a soothing male voice spoke.

"Hi!" I said enthusiastically. "My name is Christina. I found your name on a website and saw that you can treat Night Eating Syndrome?"

"Yes, I can set up an appointment with you, sure," he said.

"How long are the sessions? How much does it cost?"

"I ask for the initial session to be an hour and a half long to get a history and conduct the first treatment. The fee is $225," he said.

"Okay. That is a lot of money. I really want to stop this habit though. Have you treated a lot of patients with this problem?" I asked.

"Oh sure. Tons. It is *very* effective. Any anxiety disorder can be helped with hypnosis."

"Okay. When is your earliest appointment?"

Doug Oconnor was a tall Irish man with an even more peaceful voice in person. He hypnotized people for smoking cessation, overeating, Night Eating Syndrome — you name it. I stepped into his office with a pit in my stomach.

"So what exactly do you do?" he asked me.

"Well, I'm a pharmacy student. I go to school full-time and work for my dad."

"I meant, what are your habits?" he clarified.

"Ohhhh. Well I get up in the middle of the night and eat junk. Cookies, bread, cereal, carbs mostly. Every single night since I was 18," I said, starting to cry.

"I see. A lot of people come in for this type of thing. I can imagine it is anxiety provoking," he expressed, trying to comfort me.

I shifted in my chair and stared at the ceiling.

"Yeah. I just want to get rid of it. Is it possible to totally get rid of this?"

"I'll tell you the truth. This is a long habit that we need to break. It works in stages. Gradually we can get you to stop but it may take more than one session. How about we work on having you eat something healthy, like a piece of fruit?"

"Oh, I would love that!" I said through broken tears, wiping snot off my face with the back of my hand.

"Okay. Then let's work on that. So what I want you to do is close your eyes.... Now picture a scene somewhere in nature. A place where you feel completely safe and comfortable. Maybe it's a warm day at the beach or a rainforest and you are lying on the lush grass."

"I love the beach..." I pictured Long Beach and I started to cry. Comfort and safety were not familiar to me. The notion of this made me cry even more—I never felt safe. It was a beautiful scene.

"Okay, so you are on the beach and the sand is soft and you feel it beneath your feet. You walk down to the water's edge and peer out into the ocean. The waves are flapping up against the sand. You feel the water washing gently over your feet...then you feel the sun warming your thighs...then it moves up towards your waist...then your solar plexus....then gradually up your arms...then your whole neck and back are relaxed. Nice and relaxxxedd...." His words drifted off, slipping into the space of the room.

"Okay," he said gently, "and now I'd like you to slowly come back to your awakened state..."

I blinked my eyes open. The dim lighting felt bright to my sensitive eyes.

"How long did that feel for you?" he inquired.

"I'm not sure...a few minutes?" I said, rubbing my eyes, still half-dazed and confused.

"Great news. It was 30 minutes. The shorter it feels the better chance of it working. I will burn you a CD so you can listen to this before bed every night."

At the point after I got hypnotized, I felt my anxiety taper off. I listened to the recording of his tape every night and slowly began eating less at night. I left Doug's office feeling light, free, and boundless.

"You trust yourself and you love yourself...." He whispered in my ear each and every night, and I believed those things. I trusted myself. I loved myself.

I stopped smoking and only got up to eat a Granny Smith apple and drank a glass of water. I felt unstoppable, alert, and alive.

I learned more about the process I'd undergone. Neurolinguistic Programming (NLP) can be utilized in hypnosis, however one does not equal the other. "Neuro" through the mind, "linguistic" using language, and "programming" effecting behavior is how many hypnotherapists use hypnosis. To change a behavior, you have to change the core belief system.

I thought this treatment would be a magic bullet to cure me. Hynposis has its place in therapy for eating disorders, phobias, smoking cessation, and other conditions that involve a mind-body connection. It helped me slow down, connect with my body again, and reframe the thoughts I held about myself.

Hypnosis, NLP, mindfulness meditation, and EFT tend to change our *filter*. You experience life through a set of perceptual filters that are unique to you. Your experience is filtered first by the limits of your sensory organs: what you are able to perceive is a small slice of the world. In this sense, you are out of touch with reality, because your every perception is 'filtered' not only by your biology (for instance, 20-20 vision is about as good as it gets for humans), but also by your culture, family, education, community, and other influences from your unique personal history—teachers, mentors, friends, enemies, etc.

I'm sure you have experienced that when you change your point of view (your perception of a situation), your behavior will often change as well.

Bottom line, what you perceive determines what you get in life. If you can't see it, you can't use it, but you sure can be frustrated by what you don't perceive. These are called your "perceptual filters." Until you recognize your own filtering, you are to a large extent at the mercy of your unconscious perceptual filtering. Change your filters, and you change what you experience.

These ways of seeing things have a profound effect on how you feel and react. They come from all the beliefs and underlying assumptions that you hold in your mind, from your education, spiritual or religious training, the community you were raised in, your social status in that community, your education and teachers, your economic prosperity or poverty, your family and friends, fashions and others opinions, even TV and advertising.

The first step is to carefully examine your perceptual filtering process for what you perceive, and how you react to it.

You don't know what you don't know. Few people can easily see their world with new lenses by their own means. This is most easily done by borrowing someone else's filters to get a new perspective. It is like wearing someone else's glasses. You see things in a new way. This is why coaching is so relevant and important. If you are stuck in an area in your life but don't know why, it's because you are too close to yourself to see the problem. The coach can recognize patterns you can't see because of your own perceptual filtering. We kick and scream, because who wants to change and go into that deep uncertainty? It is so comfortable to stay where we are! But no growth will come from being certain and safe. In fact, it keeps you in destructive patterns. Sometimes God sends you wake-up calls through illness. It is up to you to listen.

Chapter 12: I've got you under my skin...

A year later I woke up sweating in a panic at two in the morning. The apartment was hot again. In the dead of winter. As my feet touched the ground of the warm apartment, I made my way to the kitchen to fetch a few of my roommate's pretzels. I hoped she didn't 1) hear me rustle through the bag, and 2) know I secretly took her food a little at a time in the middle of the night. After I retrieved some pretzels, I opened the fridge and took out a Light & Fit strawberry yogurt and fished out a metal spoon from the drawer by the microwave, then headed back to my room.

I closed the door and peeled open the purple lid, glad I was alone.

Famished, I quickly devoured the yogurt. Thoughts about residency crossed my mind. My father's tense reaction on the phone that day. My rotation presentation due in a couple of weeks. I really didn't do a thorough job on citing the article I presented that day, like my professor said.

I pushed the thoughts out of my head and went to my desk drawer. I had a peanut butter heart from Valentine's Day. I ripped open the foil and took a bite of the milk chocolate.

Only a few bites. It's a big heart.

The peanut butter overwhelmed my taste buds. I took three more bites. Then I put it away and slipped back into bed.

An hour later I got up again and went straight for my desk drawer. I couldn't leave this chocolate alone—it was staring me in the face! I couldn't throw it away, either. I would just take it out of the garbage. Ravenously, I devoured the rest of the chocolate heart.

I felt like I wanted to puke. In fact, I was going to…. An overpowering sense of nausea washed over my body. I ran to the bathroom and kneeled at the toilet, praying for the vomit to just come out already. I waited. Why wouldn't it come? I tried sticking my finger down my throat. No luck.

Fuck. Why did I eat that ENTIRE THING? What am I feeling? What don't I want to feel? I thought I was over this.

I felt shameful, nauseated, and sick. I wanted to be held and coddled like a baby. I couldn't go back to sleep now; my mind was wired and racing.

There was only one thing I could think of that would help me sleep. Walking to Kristina's room, I thought of how I could sleep through the night if someone else was next to me. I nudged her.

"Kristina. Wake up. Can I sleep in your bed tonight? I'm really anxious and I can't sleep," I whispered.

"Sure, Chris. Come in."

I had never felt so relieved. My roommate was willing to welcome me, at 2:30 in the morning, into her bed so I didn't have to be alone. I was blessed.

The next morning I was on the Q49 bus taking deep breaths. Staring up at the walls, I pictured myself running. In my daydream, there were two teams: one I used to be familiar with, another whose faces I could not make out. I knew the former team's stride, their path to follow, and who the leader was. Despite my comfort, my blood was in that team. I couldn't keep up and I didn't even want to be in the same race. I pictured myself losing my breath and withdrawing from the race all together, dissipating from view without so much as a breath to say goodbye.

"Two roads diverged in a wood and I chose to take the path less traveled by...." rang in my mind. To run with an unfamiliar team both frightened and excited me. An intuitive message came to me and I knew my stride and determination were enough to carry me. *The ties are being cut, the path is diverging, and I am on my own yet again.*

"Yo." My phone showed a text from Roy.

My stomach turned.

"What's up?" I responded.

"Call me," he wrote.

"I'm on rotations."

"What are you crazy? Trying to do a residency? Call me."

"Ugh give me 10 minutes..." I texted back. Anxiety crawled into my body as I snuck into Bellevue's 11th floor corridor and prayed for signal. AT&T service in this building literally sucked.

"Hey loser, what's goin' on?" I said, trying to break the tension.

"So Dad said you are trying to do a residency? Why don't you just work for him? You can't survive on $30,000 a year. Do you know how little that is? You can be making $120,000 a year," he said.

"I know, but I really want to try to get this residency. It's going to open up a lot of doors for me. I can survive on that amount. I have money saved..." I said, my voice wavering with doubt.

"Eh...the real world isn't like Dad's store, Christina. People are cutthroat. I'm telling you. They have no problem ratting on you or getting you in trouble. Last week one of the guys I work with did that to me. Fuckin' guy almost got me fired," he reasoned.

"Haha. Roy—I can handle it. I'm a Tarantola. Plus, I can deal with anyone," I said, convincing myself I would be okay.

"Your choice. Good luck." He hung up.

Tearing up, I slowly walked back to the computers to check patient charts for adverse drug reactions. I sniffed back the tears and pushed back the thoughts. I had a task to do—any chart that had Benadryl or Prednisone needed to be flagged and looked at to assess the cause of the allergic reaction. I wanted to crawl into a corner and cry. Or get back on the subway and go home.

"Christina, what's wrong?" Eric asked. He was a tall portly Irish man from the 11th floor pharmacy. He was absolutely ridiculous in his humor and wit and could always make me laugh.

"Eric." I paused to accentuate the gravity of the question I was about to pose. "Do you think it's possible to completely throw caution to the wind and do something that is totally against the grain for the sake of following your heart? I want to do this residency and my entire family is against it."

"I mean…residency? You'll probably end up being a clipboard. In a hospital. What type of residency would you do? And you'd be making a LOT less money than you are now. Pharmacists in retail make *bank*," he reasoned.

"I want to do an ambulatory care residency. I know there's money in retail, but will that fulfill me? I want time with my patients and I can't have time with them if I am rushing just filling their Lipitor and Singulair."

"The world is your fucking oyster! You're young, hot, going to be a PharmD! Enjoy life," he pressed, his yell turning into a whisper as we noticed other pharmacists turning from their computers to look at us.

"Yeah…guess you're right." I turned back to my empty seat. Focusing on the computer screen, I scrolled down past the listing of patients on Benadryl and Prednisone. Was this guy right? Was I just meant to play small and stay where I was comfortable? Yes, I would be making four times the amount of money if I skipped out on this residency. Roy said it too. In fact, my whole family had given me the red flag on this.

But I had a bigger vision. I had a deep feeling that what I was about to undertake was going to take gumption, strength, and courage unlike anything I'd ever endured. But I also knew what was pulsating through my veins, penetrating deep into my heart. I was a fucking Tarantola. And I was going to do a residency.

Chapter 13: I am the warrior, yes, I am the warrior, victory is mine

"How can I build my curriculum vitae?" I asked Dr. Cassagnol. A curriculum vitae is considered your "life's work" and in pharmacy we use CVs instead of resumes to document what we have done professionally. Dr. Cassagnol was my emphatic, opinionated preceptor on my month-long elective rotation at Long Island Jewish Hospital. Every morning, my partner in crime, Raquel, and I had to report to rounds with medical residents and the attending physician on the Coronary Care Unit. Rounds lasted four hours. My feet killed me despite the ever-so-classy black Crocs I wore.

"You need to get some volunteer activities under your belt. Come to Brown Bag events with me and I can help you edit your CV before Midyear in December. You are starting early, aren't you?" she asked.

"Yes. Where should I apply? Who should I talk to?" I pressed, ignoring her concern for my unrelenting need to start and finish things early.

"Well, you would probably do well in an ambulatory care setting. You can see patients and counsel them directly and have more of an impact that way. A lot of residencies out of state have those opportunities. Community pharmacy practice in New York is limited as far as what services we can offer to patients. In other states, they get reimbursed for smoking cessation counseling, diabetes education, and Medication Therapy Management."

"Okay. I'll start there. I need to really impress these people. What can I do to stand out?" I asked.

"Get business cards," she explained.

My face froze. "Well...how do I make business cards? I mean I've never done that before. Where do I start?" Anxiety crept into my mind. I had never even been on an interview — this was going to be harder than I thought.

"I'll show you," she offered. "You're such a Nervous Nelly!"

"Okay, well would you mind showing me now? I'd like to start as soon as possible."

"Sure," she said. "Let's go onto VistaPrint."

Fifteen minutes later we had a dynamic business card in 12-point Georgia font ready to print 100 copies.

That night I spent hours searching ambulatory care residencies online. I made a list of the ones that focused on volunteer opportunities, diabetes education, smoking cessation, had a focus in teaching, and could help me build leadership skills. By the end of two hours, I had a list of a dozen potential residencies, the deadlines for application submission, application requirements, and who I needed to contact for more information. I was going to make a point to call those people, I vowed. I was determined to get a residency no matter what.

Living back at home was not as easy as I thought it would be. I had moved back home after my lease expired in Queens near school. My mother was overwhelmed and frustrated with my decision to press forward and do a residency.

"How could you still want to do this to us? Don't you see you are betraying us? We *paid* for your college, Christina! Can't you just work for us for two or three years, and then do a residency?" she yelled, stomping through our kitchen, banging pots and pans around.

This was my biggest fear. Coming home to absolute chaos.

"Mom...this is my dream. I want to make an impact on the world. I want to connect with my patients and I can't do that at the pharmacy. I want to be a better pharmacist and a residency will allow me to do that."

"You won't make money. You are going to come home with $12 an hour. Dad is breaking his fucking back for you and this is how you *treat* him?!" She chucked a mustard bottle at me, barely missing my head.

"I think I need to talk to you when you are calmer..." I said, staying exactly where I was. I was afraid to move. She was too upset to think rationally.

"Yeah, I'm not *calm*. Don't worry. We'll deal with this," she replied, clomping out of the kitchen and shutting the back door. It slightly popped back open from the force.

I needed a way to process all of this; to stay in the chaos without breaking. I was not going to budge. At the risk of betraying my parents, I could not betray myself.

The pressure was too much. I felt guilty every time I walked through the door of my own home. My father's curt responses and lack of eye contact were enough to tell me he deemed this a selfish path. His energy felt dense and he barely spoke to me. My body pulsed with anxiety as the interviews for getting into a residency drew closer. Each year, residency programs and potential residency candidates met in a central location to have the first interview screening process. After a second round of interviews with a select few top candidates, each program and resident would rank their top choices, and whoever "matched" got their residency of choice. That year the annual meeting was in New Orleans. I was applying to 5 residencies out of state. My dream was to learn more about patient counseling, compounding, and diabetes care. Although I had so much passion, some days my heart raced and I sweat so much I thought I was having a panic attack. I woke up multiple times during the night, tossing and turning with fear.

I couldn't function during the day after minimal sleep. I had my primary doctor write me a prescription for 60 Xanax. She wrote it for Xanax 0.5mg and I cut them in half like she told me to so I would achieve the lowest dose. "Titrate it to the full tablet after a week if it isn't helping," she told me.

Ugh, here I am taking anxiety medication. I said I would never do this.

Yet somehow I knew I needed it to take the edge off, just to survive. I would take half a tablet at night to quell my loud mind. About 20 minutes after I split the orange tablet and popped it in my mouth, an expansive sense of relief took over me. I was able to sleep although I still got up at night to eat—and it was much worse now. Mental health had already been discussed in Drugs and Disease so I knew the mechanism of anxiolytics like Xanax, how it worked in the body and that I could develop a tolerance if I took it for a while. I used it as needed, which was pretty frequently.

I decided to attempt to quiet my mind other than popping my new best friend, Xanax. I started to take yoga classes to stay sane, connected, and grounded. There was a yoga studio a couple of towns away and I started going after work.

In my first Hatha yoga class, I gathered the multicolored wool blanket, edges frayed, and unrolled my lime green Gaiam mat. Settling into an upright position, I relaxed into the mat and brought presence to my breath.

Immediately tears came to my eyes.... A voice inside of me reminded me that this was one of the only places I now felt safe.

The instructor, Jackie, walked into the room barefoot. She unrolled her blue yoga mat and lit the incense next to the candle on the wooden shelf near the wall. Her energy was welcoming and calming. Yes, I was safe here.

She started: "In life...we tend to stuff down our emotions...so far that they wind up in our stomach...in our solar plexus..." Her voice glided along, drawing out every word and syllable. "I am going to invite you tonight...to open yourself up to express your authentic self. When you are authentic, all those around you are affected positively..."

I could drown in this woman's voice. So soothing...ready to go to sleep.

"Sometimes in life we experience...discomfort," Jackie said as she held her hands in her lap. "We can breathe through that discomfort. Invite compassion into your heart as you place your right hand gently on your beating heart," she offered. This loving kindness was so unfamiliar to me and as I placed my hand over my broken heart, the tears came. I cried in silence. I was betraying what my dad had taught me: never cry in public.

I left my problems at the door. A thought passed me like a cloud on a breezy summer day. Anxiety turned into possibility. Negativity turned into opportunity for change and growth. I realized we are always in concert with ourselves trying to find a balance; a balance between work and play, rational with emotional, stimulation and relaxation. The troublesome thoughts were revealed in the stillness, but I did not let them overwhelm me. I observed them gently and breathed into it just like Jackie told me to. I was safe in the nest of my own breath. Then, before I knew it, we were resting in *savasana*, or corpse pose. My therapy was over. Back to the chaos.

"Hey. Grab milk on your way home." A text from my father.

"Sure thing, Dad. See you soon," I replied immediately.

I pulled up to the house and paused before entering. I had to ask my father to take off to go to Midyear for my residency interview. In so few words, I had to ask for his blessing. *How will I gracefully ask him this?* I wondered. I set an intention of everything working out for everyone involved.

"Dad, I need to take off a Saturday in December for the Midyear meeting," I said carefully.

"Okay, no problem," he said sternly, focused on his paperwork.

"Okay, thanks." I turned to leave through the living room, and a feeling of extreme guilt and discomfort came over my body. That night I took another half of the orange tablet and felt the wave of anxiety diminish from my existence. That night I drifted off to sleep with my best friend Xanax....

Chapter 14: Enough is never enough...

All of my applications for residencies were mailed out in a neat package before Christmas—Ohio state, Mission Hospital, West Virginia, Brooklyn Veterans Association, and Yale-New Haven in Connecticut. I spent hours pruning the letters of intent, perfecting my curriculum vitae, arranging the three letters of recommendation, and praying I had a chance at this.

In the meantime, I was back at St. John's for my last semester of college.

I waited anxiously for a response from the 5 residencies I applied to, checking my email every day and anticipating a phone call at any moment. I hoped for a message to arrive in my inbox displaying "Residency Interview" with an enclosed invitation to fly down to North Carolina or up to Ohio.

The first email came from Ohio State with the horrible words of "We regret to inform you..." I was both shocked and in denial—I wouldn't let myself cry. *Okay, well, Ohio State wasn't my top pick anyway.*

But then West Virginia and Yale-New Haven followed suit, and the Brooklyn VA didn't bother to call or email one way or another. I still had a chance at my number one choice—Mission Hospital. In my mind I already had the interview. I visualized it, felt it, and embodied the certainty of it. After all, the director handwrote me a letter stating that I was going to make an impact on our profession and my future patients! And in reality, the other four residencies didn't hold a candle to Mission Hospital.

Then the call came.... I had just finished a Nutraceutics class in St. Albert's hall when I got a call from an 828 area code. I picked up and nervously answered.

"There have been over 75 candidates and you were number 13," said the bearer of bad news. My heart sank. They would only be interviewing 12 people this year. My heart was broken. I hung up the phone in the middle of the St. John's hallway, my friend Pete standing next to me with a look of anticipation.

"What happened?" he asked.

"I'm number 13. Lucky 13. I didn't get it...." I stifled my tears and swallowed my sadness.

He walked me to my car and hugged me. We were both in disbelief that I didn't make it to the second interview.

I went to work that day holding in my tears, pissed off that I would be stuck for another year working at the drugstore. If I were to stay, I would have to make the best of it. The wheels starting turning on potential projects I could do at Winn Drugs. I could start a diabetes education program and hold it on a Sunday. I was determined to stretch and grow as a professional even if I couldn't do a residency.

That night I ordered a book on how to be a preceptor. Maybe this would be a great opportunity. I brought up an idea of having pharmacy students at the pharmacy to assist with health fairs, to counsel patients and learn more about retail pharmacy. My sister immediately shot the ideas down; she didn't want to have to be responsible for student interns "who are lazy and know nothing." I still had a feeling it could work.

A few weeks later, I was taking notes in my Case Studies class. It was Dr. Ginzburg's class. Standing at 5 foot 4 inches, she was both intimidating and incredibly brilliant. She had dark features — her onyx eyes perfectly matched her jet-black hair. Memories of 3rd year in Alternative Medicine came to me. How she had scolded me for answering a question that was directed toward the members of the group that was presenting. I pushed my ego to the side. My mind was churning with possibility. The topic that day was Contraception and I recalled she worked out of an ambulatory clinic at Beth Israel.

During our breakout group discussions, I called her over and asked about potentially helping me edit my CV. She told me to email her and I did immediately after class. *Maybe she can help me better prepare for residency for next year. Maybe not all is lost.*

I received an email from her later that week: she wanted to meet in person to review the CV. I replied quickly and went to her office, a small cubicle in St. Albert Hall. I sat next to her desk and anxiously awaited her comments as she pulled up my CV and began scanning the document.

"Hmmm...I'm surprised you didn't get an interview. You have plenty of extracurricular and volunteer activities." She gave me some pointers on correcting my formatting and how to change the wording to enhance what I had done on my rotation experiences.

"I really wanted this, but I got denied from my five choices," I spoke with remorse.

"I understand. I'll try to think of something," She saved the changes to my CV and closed the document.

Suddenly, she turned away from the computer and I saw the light bulb go off.

"Oh wait. I forgot about Kings Pharmacy in Brooklyn. It isn't ambulatory care per se, but it's a community pharmacy residency. You will learn a lot there. I actually know the director, Dr. Chawla," she said hopefully.

"Call Dr. Chawla," she went on. "She's the director. Try to get the interview. I will email her letting her know you're interested. Maybe if they don't match this year, you can get an interview." Her onyx eyes softened in the light. I was grateful.

The Match worked like a dating service. Candidates were interviewed and the program picked their top choice. The candidates ranked their top programs and were matched up on a certain date when the results of who picked whom were revealed online.

This was my final chance. My last strike before I officially struck out. *Should I tell my father I am enrolling in this opportunity? My mother said no, what if I don't get it? I'll feel bad that I even told him and nothing came of it.*

The day the Match results came out, I was sitting in a big brown leather chair at Starbucks with a green tea on the table beside me. At 12pm the results would come out and I was praying with every last string of hope that Kings Pharmacy would appear on the computer screen. At 12:01 I scanned the list of unmatched programs, and Kings was on the list!

I dialed the number listed on the screen and left a voicemail for Dr. Chawla, stating that I knew Dr. Ginzburg and was very interested in the program. All I could do was pray and hope I would have my chance at number 6.

A few days later, I received a call from the Kings resident, Marina, offering me an onsite interview. Now the problem was telling my father I had done this. I couldn't even pretend a residency in Brooklyn meant the Brooklyn VA had invited me onsite. He would find out where I was working if I got the position—I couldn't lie. How could I approach him and tell him this? I didn't want to hurt him.

One day at work my mother started crying. She knew all the details of how I was scheduled for an interview. She must have spilled the beans to my father and wound up telling him at work of all places. I was making a cup of coffee at the Keurig machine when he approached me sounding frustrated and accusatory.

"When were you going to tell me you were applying for another residency?"

"I didn't want to tell you if there was no shot of me getting an interview. My heart isn't in it to work here, Dad." I scanned his eyes before he walked away without a word.

Still, I *had* to keep going.

Later that night, I researched the Kings website. The staff had lengthy descriptions of their titles, responsibilities, and expertise. It seemed like an amazing place that would foster all of my interests — diabetes education, being a preceptor for students, compounding, and running different clinics. Plus I would be publishing a newsletter each month focusing on how to educate patients on different health topics. It was a beautiful synchronicity and it seemed as if the universe had provided what I truly wanted.

Now it was just about nailing the interview.

Chapter 15: Cause it's the world I know...

I remember sitting in a Starbucks the day of the interview, waiting for my green tea to cool off, the steam swirling in aberrant circles. Somehow watching the steam disperse into the air calmed me a great deal. I intended to walk into the interview with poise, clarity, and passion. I knew I would wind up where I was meant to serve and I had to have faith. It wasn't easy to put myself out there once again and risk failing after being denied 5 times in a row. My deep passion and heart overrode my pride.

Walking into Kings for the first time turned out to be interesting to say the least. I approached the pharmacy counter and was greeted by an older Egyptian man, who was smiling from ear to ear.

"I'm here for the interview. My name is Christina," I said as he continued smiling at me. I read his name badge that read "Jimmy." I liked Jimmy's energy. He had kindness in his eyes that felt familiar.

"Okay. I'll get Sweta." He moved toward a door with all of the blinds closed. It felt like the scene from the Wizard of Oz with the giant curtain covering the great and powerful Oz.

Then I heard a loud male voice. "Oh no. You gotta be fuckin' kiddin' me."

I turned my head to the left where the "Pick up" window was. The mystery voice was shielded by the huge partition walling off the pharmacists and techs from the outside counter space.

Oh Lord…what am I in for? I thought to myself as I chuckled. My tension eased.

Finally, I was summoned by Marina, the kindhearted resident I had spoken to over the phone.

I entered the office and sat down with Dr. Chawla and Marina. Dr. Chawla was a beautiful Indian woman with large eyes that reminded me of an owl. She wore a white lab coat and sat across from me. Dr. Chawla explained the structure of the interview. She would explain the program, interview me, and take a tour with Marina. Then I would complete a mock counseling session with her and answer basic pharmacy calculations.

She brought out a black binder labeled "Residency Structure" and explained the nature of what I'd be responsible for, how each facet of the residency would work.

A community pharmacy residency has goals and objectives the resident must complete to graduate. Much of it was a blur as I zoned out in anticipation for the interview questions. I nodded most of the time, pretending I was comprehending and processing this new information.

I tuned back in when she started asking questions.

"What have you done in the past when someone superior to you has embarrassed you in front of a patient?"

Quick, try to think of a different answer. Should I not get too deep into the dysfunction of my family dynamic?

"I don't think I've ever really had that happen," I lied. *Shit, I have such a bad poker face.*

"You can't think of a time when someone made you look bad?" She had sensed my lie buried beneath the layers of pain I tried to hide.

"Well, I worked with my sister and there were times I've had to take her in the back and ask her how we can resolve the issue at hand," I said. Little did she know how my sister degraded me, hid work from me, and delegated to me the tasks she didn't think were fit for a pharmacist. I recalled her saying, "I shouldn't have to call this insurance company. You do it." And telling a customer, "I would never want to go to Italy—it's so dirty!" when she knew I was planning my trip there. None of that mattered now. *Suppress it, Christina. This isn't the time to bring that up.*

The questioning went on for a while. Dr. Chawla asked about ideas I had to improve patient care, why I became a pharmacist, and why I was a good candidate. Every so often I would glance at the various certificates and pledges on the wall of the office. CERTIFIED DIABETIC EDUCATOR embossed in stunning Segoe script. Oath of a Pharmacist. That oath—so near and dear to my heart. I remembered reciting it at my White Coat ceremony in 3rd year of school and feeling like it was my wedding vow, tears welling up in my eyes with each word.

Finally the questions were over and I felt like I had responded with clarity and certainty.

After Marina showed me around the pharmacy, we passed Lenny, one of the technicians, and made small talk with him. Immediately, I matched the previously overheard profanity with his voice. I had a feeling he was going to be my favorite if I got the job. He seemed like a warmhearted, gentle giant who would give great life advice.

Dr. Chawla came to retrieve me and led me to take my test. I sat in a small room with a long table covered in books and junk. Supposedly they were cleaning up from an audit. I looked at the first page of the test — easy calculations. Amoxicillin dose conversion mg/kg, mL/min to gtt/hr. All basic pharmacy math I'd learned in the first few years of school. I double checked the calculations and confidently turned the page.

The next page was a prescription for Lisinopril 5mg, a blood-pressure medication, and it stated that the patient wanted Claritin-D for her allergies. I was to mock counsel Dr. Chawla on how to properly take the medication. The patient was 32 years old and of child-bearing age. Lisinopril is an ACE inhibitor, which is contraindicated in pregnancy. In fact, it is teratogenic — meaning it can disturb the development of an embryo or fetus, especially in the 3rd trimester. *Do I mention that when I counsel? Let's get some other points in there — ACE-induced cough, orthostatic hypotension; avoid pseudoephedrine from the Claritin-D because it may increase blood pressure and heart rate.* I jotted my ideas on a blank sheet of paper and prayed I had done everything right.

I realized just how long the interview had run; I still had to go to work in Kings Park that day.

"I need to go to work," I explained to Marina. "I'm really sorry." I still had to complete the mock counseling on the Lisinopril prescription with Dr. Chawla. I completed the counseling session from memory since I had left my paper in the other room. I felt confident as I completed the counseling session.

I said goodbye to everyone and stepped out into the sunlight on Flatbush Avenue.

I called Pete, who had been waiting for me and driving around Prospect Park. While I waited for him, Dr. Chawla walked by on her way back from grabbing lunch and approached me.

"Is someone picking you up?"

I noticed a change in her disposition. It was less formal, even friendly. Her energy was different.

"Yes, my friend Pete. He's driving around and coming back to the pharmacy now. Thank you for everything," I said with a smile.

I left Kings that day with the fate of my future in the hands of this woman who was a complete stranger to me. I kept positive thoughts in my mind, reiterating to myself how well the interview went.

The next 2 days were torture as I calculated my fate at my father's store. How could I leave my family after my father had trained me for 10 years since I was a young girl? He had been my inspiration, my guide along this journey. He was the one who inspired me to be a pharmacist in the first place. He would quiz me on our half-hour car rides to work.

"What are the three signs of diabetes?" he'd asked. "Remember the three Ps, Christina. Polyuria, polydypsia, polyphagia." He had quizzed me on brand and generic names of medication before I even got into pharmacy school. I had observed him interact with ease as he spoke to patients in the pharmacy. He was the entire reason why I was so comfortable talking to anyone, stranger or not. I was grateful for those lessons and yet I knew I couldn't stay. My heart told me I was destined to make a big impact in this world, and I could not turn away from that.

Chapter 16: If you leave me now, you'll take away the biggest part of me. Ohhhh baby, please don't go...

I was to be expecting the phone call from Dr. Chawla on a Thursday evening. The time was passing by as I was typing prescriptions at the pharmacy—3:00, 5:00, 5:30. No call. My heart started sinking. *Did they forget? Was it a bad or good sign that I wasn't getting a call? Surely it was good – they were calling the other candidate to tell them the regretting news. Or was it bad because they didn't want to have to call and hear my groan over the phone as they denied me?* My mind kept vacillating in the background as I tried my best to focus on filling prescriptions.

Finally my cell phone rang.

I hurried into the back room to accept the call.

"Hello?" I answered nervously.

"Hi Christina, it's Dr. Chawla. Sorry to get back to you so late. We have good news for you...." A wide smile broadened across my face. "We want to invite you to come work with us," she offered.

"Yes!! Thank you. Sure," I said, trying to subdue my voice. My dad was in the other room, for Christ's sake.

"You sound very calm about it," she said, curious as to why I wasn't jumping for joy and screaming like I was on Nitro at Six Flags.

"Oh, I'm sorry. I am at work and didn't want to be too loud." A feeling of guilt came over me. I couldn't rejoice and go screaming down the aisles.

"I will be sending you a contract in the mail to sign and return to us. Also, I'm not sure if you need to sign up for your board exams. We also wanted you to come in for training in June. You don't have to come on consecutive days, just whenever you are free. I am sure you'll want to celebrate with your friends and family."

Ha. Yes, I'm sure the family will be thrilled, I thought as I thanked her and hung up.

Then it dawned on me: I was officially leaving Winn Drugs.

A million thoughts raced through my mind. *How will I tell my father without hurting him? Should I not tell him now? How will I fare working in another pharmacy for a year? As a new pharmacist?* I finally got what I really wanted—a residency. A chance to spend time actively learning, deepening relationships with patients, and becoming more familiar and comfortable with having the huge responsibility that comes with being a pharmacist.

It took every ounce of courage to knock on my father's wooden door. I held my breath and waited for him to speak.

"Come in," he responded as I opened the door a crack. He had his eyes focused on the ceiling with his hands behind his head, leaning back in his black chair. His eyes suddenly met mine and I noticed the sadness in them and the dark bags under his big eyes from lack of sleep. My mother made sure to tell me he hadn't been sleeping the past couple of weeks.

"Dad. I got the residency," I said slowly, each syllable harder to speak than the one before.

"Congratulations," he said, forcing the word out. "When do you start?"

"July first."

"Good for you." He turned back to his paperwork.

I went back to work. I could count the hundreds of times we had carpooled and he had driven me to and from work. My mother had taken his car home that day. I had to drive my father home when the gates closed. Now *I* was in the driver's seat. The eerie symbolism sent chills down my spine. The tension was so thick I heard every syllable of noise. The click of a seatbelt. The beat of my own heart. I just kept my hands at 10 and 2 hoping he wouldn't jump over the center console and choke me to death.

He tried asking questions about the residency — what I would be doing, activities, where I would live, how I would commute. But deep down, I knew he was at the edge of frustration, the cusp of an internal breakdown. His energy dug deep down into my soul and guilted me to the core.

I didn't know how else to tell him I couldn't work in an environment where I felt threatened by my own family, where I knew I would never grow into the professional I wanted and needed to become. I couldn't find the words to express how much I wanted to make an impact on my future patients, despite a mere salary of $38,000. It didn't matter; no consolation would have helped at that point. He had always been a black-and-white thinker and this situation was no different. I had betrayed them in the worst way. If I wasn't on their team, I was against them.

At a stoplight, I texted my mother. She had been hot and cold lately, but I thought she would be proud of me for getting what she knew I truly wanted.

"Mom, I got the residency!!!"

I didn't have much time to dwell on how guilty I felt or how excited I was for this new chapter to begin. I had an exam to study for the next day. I packed up my book-bag and headed to my friend Brittany's to focus on studying.

As I traveled to Brittany's house, I felt a sigh of relief that I was finally free. Now I could grow and learn my own way on my own terms. I would live in Brooklyn somewhere near the residency. What was in Brooklyn, anyway? Aside from the Brooklyn Bridge, I hadn't ventured out there. I would worry about that after the exam—Britt and I had to study.

As it turned out, my mom wasn't keen on the news I delivered through text. The first text I received was about how I was a "horrible, back-stabbing daughter" and "could finally get away from my dysfunctional family." *Okay, she is upset.* But then the texts came in droves—"You aren't my daughter anymore. I'm not coming to graduation. You fucked us royally. After all we did for you. We took you out to dinners with David. We paid for your college. We gave you an apartment!"

Guilt. Grief. Nausea. I wanted to puke. Suddenly the amicable, sweet, and nurturing woman I had known my whole life had become a rage-filled demon. It was such a heavy-weighted sensation to feel as if the safety blanket of everything I had ever known was being pulled from underneath me.

Fuck. I'm trying to concentrate now.... How can I concentrate for the Nutraceutics exam while my phone is being blown up with hateful text messages?

"Chris, just ignore it. Let's keep studying. How many calories per gram does a fat have?" Brittany asked, our usual question-and-answer banter.

"Nine..." I said reflexively, my voice trailing off to meet my terror somewhere along the way.

I could barely talk but there wasn't really a choice here; the exam was in 12 hours. I texted Pete and felt like dying. Pete drove right from work to comfort me and we started talking about my parents and the argument that had sparked the biggest fight of my life.

"I can see where they're coming from," he responded, always neutral. My stomach dropped and it was questionable if my dinner would stay down after this conversation. The angry text messages from my mother came in heaps and I wondered when they would end.

"Guys, I feel so sick…"

Brittany turned to me and said, "You know what we need? A SHOT! Let's celebrate, Chris. You got a residency!!!"

"I'm down," I said without hesitation. I didn't want to feel anymore. It was unbearable. And of course Pete was ready for alcohol on a Thursday night. Brittany carried out the Georgi peach vodka from her back room and set it in front of me. We got red Solo cups and toasted to my accomplishment, to this long journey full of sweat and tears. Mostly tears. To me the toast meant so much more — it represented my courage, hard work, and resilience. I took a hard swallow followed by the Capri sun chaser. *Life is sweet after all.*

"Let's go to Massapequa. We can go to McGorey's," Brittany squealed.

"Yeah, fuck it. Let's go," I agreed. The rest of the night was a blur.

Chapter 17: Ha ha ha ha, stayin' alive. Stayin' alive.

Bzzzzz. Bzzzzz.

I felt the vibration of my cell phone underneath my warm body as I slowly stirred awake.

Cotton mouth. Pulsating headache. Anxiety. Pete was still sleeping on the couch.

What time is it? Where am I? Oh yeah, Brittany's house.

As I rolled over to read the texts from my phone, I regretted every sip of alcohol I had ingested the night prior.

I read the texts from my mother: "I am throwing all of your stuff into the garage. You better come get it," she wrote.

I jumped up as my mouth fell open. A rush of blood went to my head. *Ugh – hangover headache.*

"Britt, I have to go. My mom is throwing me out of my house..." My voice trailed off as I grabbed a bottle of water from the counter.

Pete and I pulled up to my house and I saw a shoe fly out of the front door as my mother appeared on the porch.

"Oh nice. You bring Pete with you?! You selfish bitch. You ruined us," she shouted from the deck.

She began going in and out of the house throwing items outside one by one. Shoes, coats still clinging to the hangers, jewelry — anything and everything that I had culminated and possessed over the past 23 years.

Fuck, I need my Xanax.

"Pete, try to ask to go into the house. I think I have some Xanax left," I begged him to approach the door.

"You aren't allowed inside. Stay the fuck away from this door. Oh, and you see this picture?" She motioned to the picture I kept on my nightstand of my father holding me as a 3-year-old in the pool.
"THIS...means nothing," she said as she smashed the frame onto the deck, breaking the glass into a million pieces.

Luckily my tiny orange best friend Xanax had already been tossed out into the mix of the mound of clothes and totes. I spotted the prescription bottle with my name embossed on the vial. I prayed to God there were pills left. Uncapping the amber vial, I saw *one* tiny, oval, orange pill. *Lord help us all. One pill left.* I popped it in my mouth without any water and took a deep breath.

Next my father came outside. His face was cold and stoic as he approached me.

"Give me the keys to the drugstore," he demanded.

I slowly reached into my bag and took off the gold key that unlocked the gate for the store. I lowered my eyes as he walked back toward the house. Shame, guilt, and sadness washed over me. I had let them down by choosing to do a residency instead of work at their pharmacy. And this was my punishment.

As the Xanax began to take effect, my heart expanded. I was calm and centered in a way I hadn't been before. I fully believe God was there that day, surrounding me with love. I was safe amongst the chaos.

As Pete and I quietly gathered my clothes, shoes, jewelry, and dignity into his car, I knew that someday I would tell this story. I *knew* in the deepest part of me that I had a bigger purpose to fulfill and I could not stay at my father's pharmacy. I had to take control of my own life and it was worth any amount of emotional, mental, or physical pain to get there.

There is something that happens deep inside of you when you are at the bottom. It is a scary, uncertain place to be uprooted from your home, to be jobless and to completely surrender, hoping the universe will catch you. My body pulsed with fear and adrenaline. I was in survival mode. Yet I had faith that somehow I would survive.

The closest person I could think of to go to was my Aunt Grace, who lived a couple of towns away. Pete and I trucked bags full of my belongings to my Aunt Grace's. After 3 roundtrips back and forth from my former house to my aunt's, I realized how much baggage I had—figuratively and physically. I spread out my clothes to be folded on my aunt's table when this reality sunk in. It was a mess. I was a mess, but I stayed focused.

We put my clothes into vacuum-sealed bags to conserve space so it could all fit into my car. I was torn apart but I had no choice but to focus on the solutions. I was already planning out my next job, my goals for finding an apartment, and moving my money from the bank near my father's pharmacy. I didn't have time to process what was really going on and all of the levels of pain that were striking every cell in my body.

"I'm sorry, honey, but I can't let you sleep here. Your dad just texted me and said if I let you stay, he'll be mad at me. I really shouldn't get involved in your fight," my aunt said, and the shock hit me.

What the fuck? Why is this happening?

I slept at Brittany's house again that night. I had time to calm down during the day and forced myself to laugh about it by taking a picture next to my packed-out car. Hair dryers, jeans, shoes, makeup, towels, pillows, bank statements, and picture frames crowded my tiny Mazda 3. I needed to find an apartment ASAP because Brittany's mom understandably didn't want to get involved either, nor have me become a squatting duck in her basement. Her family was in disbelief of what had happened to me. To be truthful, I was too.

I called my old internship job to see if they had any available openings and got a job the next day. I needed an apartment too. I resorted to the free WiFi at Starbucks and it was my lifesaver as I searched Craigslist for potential apartments. I called a few listings and was scheduled to go look at an apartment later in the week. It didn't seem soon enough though.

Later that day I drove to Pete's house in Howard Beach. Pete's mom pulled out the housing listings from the Queens Chronicle. I sat cross-legged on Pete's white couch to search the paper for ads. A big ad popped out at me—**Studio apartment in Lindenwood $1000/month. Call Fred**.

"Lindenwood is a nice area," Pete's mom said. "It's right up the block. You should go look at it today!"

I called the broker and was allowed to view the apartment that same day. Fred was an older Italian gentleman with a distinct hooked nose who smelled of cigarettes, had yellow teeth and a raspy voice. As he unlocked the first-floor door, I was immediately impressed. The cherry wood cabinets in the kitchen looked pristine and the bathroom tiles were gorgeous. The prior tenant had left a dresser with four drawers that I could use.

"I love it!" I exclaimed and Pete agreed it was a reasonably priced apartment.

"Okay it's yours. You can move in in two weeks," Fred responded.

Over those following 2 weeks that I considered myself "homeless" in jocularity, I came to a deeper appreciation for the simple things in life. I felt a deep sense of gratitude for my resourcefulness. I had a temporary job until July 1 when my residency would start. For two weeks I stayed with Liz, a girl I had met on one of my CVS rotations. She was eclectic, free-spirited, and refreshingly open. She reminded me of myself in so many ways and I was fortunate to be able to stay at her second-floor apartment in West Hempstead. Distraught and heartbroken, I poured out my pain and Liz listened with compassion.

"Oh honey, I'm sorry. Let's meditate. We can even get you a rose quartz stone from A Time for Karma. It's a cute little place in Rockville Center. You'll love it," she offered. I felt safe again.

One of the first nights at Liz's apartment, she put on a YouTube video with calming music and guided me through a meditation. As we listened to the gentle harmony of the harp, she told me to relax, focus on breathing, and pretend I was floating freely in the night sky. I had never felt so grateful to have a friend. When everything was gone, all I had were my belongings packed into my car and this girl who I barely knew but who had graciously allowed me into her home.

Even though I had an apartment, I had virtually nothing going into it. During that time Liz took me to the dollar store on Hempstead Turnpike to find glassware and kitchen mugs, plates, and bowls. I had money saved, but who knew how long that would last me. The residency wasn't starting for another 3 months and I needed all of the basics just to function in my new apartment. We did the best we could to buy only the necessary items, and because Liz was a savvy bargain shopper, it made it so much easier. She spent all day with me at Target pruning over decorations, Swiffers, and groceries for my new home. Most importantly, she made me feel accepted on this journey.

At the end of that long day of shopping, I felt satisfied that slowly but surely, my apartment was becoming a home. The only thing missing was a bed. I needed to get the full-sized bed from my house in Copiague. I asked my father to let me use the truck to transport the bed to Howard Beach.

"Find another way. Rent a U-haul. You can't use the truck."

I would have to do it the hard way.

The U-haul place in Copiague was the closest one, but was hardly a sight to see. Pete and I walked in and I was in complete disgust. The floor was so heavily covered in junk you couldn't even see the bottom of the floor, which took on a new shade of black after years of abuse and lackluster cleaning. The owner was a sluggish, heavyset man who had papers strewn all over his desk. I found it hard to trust such a person, especially since he quoted one price over the phone and the tables turned the minute I stepped into that dump. I reluctantly handed the owner my credit card as a questionable cat jumped onto a pile of papers.

Oh Lord, how does this happen to me? I signed the receipt and we headed to my house in Copiague. Or what I used to call my house.

No one was home, but I felt like a trespasser as I unlocked the door to the place I'd known for 23 years. Every step felt weighted and sharp, like I was walking on glass. As we approached what used to be my old room, my mouth fell open. They had knocked down the wall that connected my room to the dining room. The ceiling fan and light fixtures were removed, the television and L-shaped, cream-colored desk and dressers had vanished. My entire childhood room was gutted, stripped, and exposed. I felt a deep sinking feeling in my stomach. This was my dad's way of controlling the situation—by ridding evidence that I ever existed.

As we dissembled my bed and carried the mattress out, I took one last look at my empty room. All that was left was some debris, dirt, and four depressions in the rug where the legs of my bed used to be. Just as we were loading the mattress into the truck, my mom came home.

"Yeah, Dad didn't want to leave the TV in your room for you to have. We took it away," she said. *They are still trying to punish me.* The guilt was deep enough to drown in.

My apartment finally felt whole as Pete and I assembled and made my bed, tucking in the soft grass green-colored sheets and placing the pillows at the head of the bed. Some sort of *physical* normalcy existed for a brief period of time.

While I was waiting to move into the new apartment, I was still living with Liz and busting my ass working three days a week and still finishing up my last semester in pharmacy school. The anticipation of graduating eased my sadness, dulling the pain of being separated from my family. On the mornings I had work, I would trek out to my Mazda 3 and sift through the clear plastic leaf bags to search for a matching outfit to wear. I had too many bags of clothes to fit in Liz's studio apartment.

After locating a matching outfit, I'd travel to Town Total in Melville, which was about 45 minutes away. I'd select a cubicle near the front of the office and prepare to counsel patients on their medication. I conducted Medication Therapy Management sessions, a phone-based service provided by Medicare Part D plans to their patients in order to minimize long-term costs (hospitalizations, doctor visits, etc.) and to ensure a patient was compliant and on the optimal drug therapy for their condition.

We used a computer-based platform to view the patient's medications and, prior to calling them, assessed what conditions they might have and if they were on the right medications for their condition based on clinical guidelines. The calls were commission-based: the more calls you made, the bigger your paycheck would be. There was such a fierce drive in me. I hit a record for making the most calls out of everyone in the office.

As I moved into my apartment, I realized how alone I really was. Liz was all the way in Hempstead and I didn't have close friends in this new area. At night I would meditate. It helped relieve some of the tension, but my moods fluctuated significantly. I would buy peanut butter, cereal, and cookies, eating to numb the residual pain. I couldn't keep those foods in my house because I had no self-control. Chunky peanut butter was always my biggest trigger to overeat, my drug of choice.

It didn't feel right in my body to hold that kind of anger and resentment. But I also had no idea how to clear that away. *How can I let this go? How can I lessen the pain that digs deep into my heart?* I decided to continue praying for guidance, meditating, and going to hot yoga as those things seemed to calm my internal storm. I would come home from work at night and sit on my tile floor with a scented candle. The glow of the candle soothed me and lit up the darkness of the room. Closing my eyes, I would focus only on my breath. Then the thoughts would come.

"Yeah—you go be happy. We'll take care of this," the terse voice from my mom screamed at me.

Stop thinking about anything. Relax the mind; that was in the past.

I'd picture my parents and the fine lines that grew on their faces since all of this started. Guilt. Fear. Abandonment.

FOCUS ON THE BREATHING. In and out. Come on, Christina.

When everything got quiet, the tears would fall. They were thick tears, but it felt good to release the emotions that still had such a strong grip on me. I just kept breathing...

Chapter 18: I gotta feeling that tonight's gonna be a good night

My graduation day came. On a warm, sticky spring night, I found myself at Liz's apartment. Liz closed the lid of her toilet and sat me down so she could do my makeup.

"You have such big, gorgeous eyes. They're so easy to apply makeup to," she said as I smiled, excited and nervous for what was to come that night in the auditorium.

As she swirled the brush into the cream-colored palette, my mind drifted off to the reality of how important this day was for me. I had struggled for a year to get a residency. It was all I had wanted and it was now my source of both pain and pleasure. I was so proud of my endurance, my strength, and commitment to making my needs a priority in my own life. Yet I was ashamed for betraying my family. For so long, I'd been controlled, directed and molded by my father. Not only was he the biggest influence in my life, he had become my biggest enemy over the past year. Despite what my mother said about not coming to graduation, my parents were coming along with my grandmother and my Aunt Grace.

Will they be proud of me? Will they applaud when I walk across the stage? What if they don't even care? All I wanted was for them to say, "Good job. We are so proud of you."

I took a deep breath as Liz finished my blush. She knew I liked my cheeks to be a light rosy pink. I thanked her and got dressed by the air-conditioner, slipping on my black heels and my half-white half-beige ruffled dress.

"You look beautiful, sweetheart. I'll see you later at the ceremony!" She gave me a hug before I left for St. John's.

Carneseca Arena was filled with red caps and gowns. Familiar faces caught my eye as I walked through the hallway down to the roped-off area for us graduates. A well of anxiety, sadness, and joy hit me, exploding like a stuffed piñata. I couldn't let myself fall to pieces. As my classmates filtered into the room, I smiled and took pictures with them. I told my friends they looked beautiful and congratulated everyone I saw. I was my hyper, enthusiastic self, like I was supposed to be on the outside — but inside I was lonely. Inside I was dying.

Soon enough, Dean Brocavich lined us up alphabetically and prepared for us to enter the main room of the gym. My mood shifted as I walked confidently into the gym, scanning the crowd for my parents. I spotted Aunt Grace and Grandma, although my grandmother couldn't spot me as my aunt tried to point to me. They were sweet for coming.

After we found our seats, the ceremony began with the National anthem as I saw my parents take a seat next to my sister and her husband. All of the pharmacy professors were seated on stage. It was if they were supporting us all and witnessing this transformational event.

Then the keynote speaker, Dean Barone, took the stage. Dean Barone began speaking about how he never expected to become Dean of Rutgers University. He was raised by Italian parents who pushed him to excel and when he decided to do a residency, they couldn't understand. *Why would he take such a pay cut? What was a residency anyway?* My mouth literally dropped open.

He spoke about controlling your own destiny, not allowing other people to be in command of your life. He spoke about going with your gut feeling when making a decision. My throat choked up and my heart swelled. Each word out of this man's mouth resonated with me.

One of my classmates whispered to me, "Wow it's like he's talking to you."

I simply nodded as I wiped away the tears and looked into the crowd at my parents. After he spoke, I clapped loudly and looked back at Pete, who was smiling at me. We made a silent acknowledgement of the truth of what this man just spoke of and I turned my attention back to the stage.

It was finally time for us to receive our diplomas and walk across the stage to be hooded by Dean Mangione. I nervously awaited my turn, looking for Liz's exuberant smile to the right of the stage. I couldn't see her so I kept inching my way up, following the flow of the line and the people in front of me.

As I approached the stage, I saw one of my professors, Dr. Arya, take out her camera and wave to me. I was surprised to see tears in her eyes. Her expression melted the tears from mine.

"Dr. Christina Tarantola," Dean Brocavich announced.

I walked onto the stage, taking each step gracefully, being careful not to trip. My eyes met with Dean Mangione, the man with a heart of gold who I had come to know and trust over the past 6 years. I shook his hand and turned to face the crowd as he placed the black hood around my shoulders. I was overwhelmed with a radiating happiness and level of ecstasy I had never experienced. I thanked him and felt the tears seeping down my face as I walked to my seat. I was trying so hard to hold onto the feeling. But just like Adrienne had taught me—feelings are temporary, and that feeling fleeted just as quickly as it came.

Chapter 19: I feel like dancin' dancin' dance the night away

After graduation, I needed to start studying for my board exams. I had passed compounding in January but still had the MJPE and NAPLEX exams to pass. But first, I took some time to have fun and get out of my head for a while.

Liz and I drove around listening to *bachata* music. I loved the rhythm of the music as it swelled in the speakers of her '98 grey Toyota on our way to satiate ourselves with cheap eat Dominican food off Hempstead Turnpike. We were both broke, but the *chicharrón* and crispy *tostones* filled our bellies. Liz was a regular there and she spoke beautiful Spanish to the cooks.

"Hola, mi negra! Como estas? Dos chicharrón, por favor," she said. The "r" rolled off her tongue and smoothly carried through the air as I took in the sounds. I reveled in the fluidity of the arcane language. The melody of Romeo Santos, a famous bachata singer, hummed on the radio behind the grill.

"Oh my God, Chris! I want to see Romeo Santos so badly. This guy from Brooklyn is *totally* into me and he said he could get me a VIP pass to sit front row at his concert next month. Want to come?!"

"Um, sure," I said, moving my hips in sync with the music. Liz grabbed my hands and led me in the bachata dance. Her finesse in dancing trumped mine, but I let go and sank into the syncopation of the music.

"I love bachata music, Liz...I want to sign up for classes somewhere," I said.

"Yes, do it! It's so ironic because you'd think these songs are happy based on the beat, but they are actually songs about heartbreak and lost love," she explained, twirling me in front of the glass encasement of *empanadas*.

Love. Well, my dear, I've learned that love is lost.

Later that week, I signed up for weekly bachata classes at Lorenz Latin dance studio in Glendale, Queens. I knew no one there. I didn't care. I wanted to feel free, alive, and like myself again. I needed to dance again.

The dance studio resembled what I was used to—glass mirrors and wooden floors, but there was a set of stairs for extended dance space in the rear of the studio. I was confident I could learn quickly and I just wanted to get started dancing. The instructor was a tall thin Dominican man. He smiled, yet had a firm look on his face like he meant business.

"We are going to start slow and build on the steps. Some of you are beginners and some are completely new."

We started with basic steps: right foot step to the right, left foot meets it. Left foot step to the left, right foot meets it. I swayed my hips easily with the staccato beat along with the other students. Looking around at the other people in the class, I felt connected.

They were learning with me, misstepping at times and tripping over their feet.

We formed pairs and I linked hands with a complete stranger, our fate decided by the classroom positioning. My partner was a tall Spanish man with dark penetrating eyes. He gripped my hand as the music started and I followed the choreography, faltering on one step as I contemplated how sexy his masculine energy was. *Damn....* He placed his right hand on my hip for the routine and led me into a turn. I melted into his lead and met his gaze. We finished the routine and switched partners. Fog had formed on the mirrors and I caught myself smiling at my own reflection. I felt free, sexy, feminine, connected, and for a split second, desired by this stranger. Most importantly, I felt *alive* again.

Like this and so many times before, Liz had always made me feel better. She was spunky, a free spirit, and compassionate. She'd come over the night before my 24th birthday, and we drank red wine from my dollar-store glasses and talked, laughed, and enjoyed the randomness of our Monday night meet-up. She had surrounded me with love, and that was enough.

I didn't expect anything from my parents anymore, not even for my birthday that year. However, my father surprised me with a present. It was wrapped in a recycled grocery-store paper bag and was in the shape of a book. I peeled back the paper and saw the book I had been talking about over the past couple of weeks. *The Alchemist.*

"Thanks, Dad, this means a lot," I said hugging him, feeling the stiffness of his reciprocal embrace.

"Sure, no problem," he replied.

I couldn't wait to read it. I'd heard of the book through Dr. Chawla and it had come up in conversation at another point at Town Total, the place I worked after Winn Drugs but before my residency. Every morning I would dig into a chapter as I rode the A train to work. As I uncovered more of the story, I realized how ironic it was that my father had given me this very book just before I would start my residency on July 1st. The story was so closely related to the events that were happening in my life.

The protagonist, Santiago, rebels against his father's wishes of being a priest and instead wants to travel the world to seek his Personal Legend. "Everything you could want is in our village. Why would you want to leave? The prettiest women are here, the best land," the father argues. But the boy still wants to travel, so he becomes a shepherd. The boy is seeking his "personal legend," or purpose in life. This was strangely aligned to my journey of courage and attempting to find my own purpose. It was so clear to me that I was absolutely guided and supported by the universe. And I couldn't help but think that the universe conspires to bring you closer to your deepest desires.

My first week at Kings Pharmacy flew by. One day, Marina had to compound Total Parenteral Nutrition orders and I volunteered to go with her. Kings had a huge clean room for compounding sterile products. She shadowed me as I typed in the four orders and then gowned up to compound.

"So you'll have enough FreeAmine, D5, and sterile water," she said, implying I was doing this alone.

A flash of fear came over me and quickly dissipated. I wasn't scared—I knew my memory served me well and I had shadowed Marina plenty of times before. I gowned up, putting blue booties on my feet, a hair cover, yellow over-cover, a mask, and gloves. I wheeled the silver cart into the IV room and made sure to take my time. Two bags had insulin and all 4 had multivitamin, which I added at the end. I put my Pandora on and got to work, calibrating the load cell of the IV machine, priming and verifying each ingredient, and spraying the vial tops with alcohol. As I added the insulin, I realized how careful I had to be as a pharmacist. An excess of insulin could cause low blood sugar, coma, and even death. I had to pay close attention to detail and ensure everything was exactly right.

An hour later, as I placed the 6 finished IV bags into a gallon-sized Ziploc bags, I felt accomplished. This was such a unique experience. I was improving my range of skills during residency. I thought to myself, *When you take a leap of faith, there are endless possibilities to be discovered.*

Sharing an office made me realize how much I really absorbed the energy of other people. Dr. Chawla's presence in our office threw me off, especially if she came in with an irritated energy. I wasn't sure how to explain the energy shift when she walked in, but I noticed my upper back would tighten. She had dozens of framed certificates and degrees hanging by her desk, and pictures of her traveling to different areas of the world on various trips and excursions. She had visited 35 countries in her life and travel was a staple for her, not a luxury. Being a professor at Long Island University gave her the freedom of having 5 weeks off during the summer. I both admired her and feared her.

Despite all of that, we wound up having several meaningful conversations. Somehow our conversations would shift into talking about all of the self-help gurus—Caroline Myss, Deepak Choprah, Eckhart Tolle. She would tell me about her weekly meeting at the Open Center with a medical intuitive, a term I hadn't heard before. She introduced me to the idea of the chakras, or energy centers that run down the centerline of the body. If they were out of balance or blocked, it could lead to energy stagnation and disease in the body. The medical intuitive can see impressions of where these blockages are in the person and identify ways to self-heal. This concept was so interesting to me that I decided to Google medical intuition, Caroline Myss, and energy healing. I couldn't help but believe I had something to learn from this and maybe, just maybe, this would be my path to healing.

I would watch Caroline Myss on YouTube explaining "Why people don't heal." I got lost in her words; they seemed to speak directly to me. I learned about the seven chakras of the body and grew to know them by heart. Those seven energy centers became the language I recited over in my mind as I tried to understand my own disease.

There are seven power centers in your body, called "chakras." The state of each chakra reflects the health of a particular area of your body. It also reflects your psychological, emotional, and spiritual well-being. Every thought and experience you've ever had gets filtered through these chakra databases. Each event is recorded into your cells. In other words, *your biography becomes your biology.*

When chakra energy is blocked or congested, emotional and physical illness can arise. "People don't heal because if they hold onto the pain and show you their wounds, you'll understand and feel sympathy for them. Wounded people attract other wounded people," Caroline Myss reasoned. She believed disease was not just about nutrition, but how we invest our energy into our past. You drain yourself of life-force energy if you keep the past alive. Clinging to your wounds becomes the reason you don't heal.

It made so much sense. Think about it: when a baby cries, it gets attention. If it is sick, it gets extra love and attention. Unconsciously, some people as adults cling to their wounds to get love and attention. It requires other people to constantly ask, "How are you feeling? How are you doing?" Most people don't want to admit this, but this is the reality of unconscious beliefs. *If I stay sick, I will get love.* These are maladaptive ways of getting love that were learned in childhood. These ways do not serve us as adults. There are other ways to give and receive love that do not involve compromising your body, mind, or spirit.

The stress-diathesis model is a psychological theory that states that we are all vulnerable to illness in a certain area in our body. When we are stressed, it triggers that illness to come alive, so to speak. Also known as a biological predisposition, wherever that vulnerable area is will start exhibiting symptoms.

My weak spot was my stomach and even as a child I had stomach pain from anxiety. I realized that my solar plexus chakra was blocked, meaning I gave my power away to others instead of harnessing it for myself. Undercharged or blocked solar plexus chakra manifested as low self-esteem and lack of personal power, resulting in eating disorders, weight gain, diabetes, and issues with other organs near that area two inches above the navel. I was fascinated and yet held back by these destructive patterns.

This is all well and good — but *how do I heal?* I wondered. Soon I was on a mission again--this time with the determination to heal.

Chapter 20: Now I know I've got to...run away

Even though I was becoming aware of my patterns and where my energy was blocked, I was miserable. During the day at my residency I would get easily frustrated if I couldn't fix a problem or if I was trying to delegate a task and someone wasn't respecting me. I was emotionally triggered by someone with authority telling me what to do because it reminded me of my father. Those wounds were fresh and it felt caustic to accept orders from someone when I wanted so desperately to be "free" and independent.

One day Dr. Chawla sat me down and talked to me about having more input in the pharmacy.

"I notice you are reluctant to voice your opinion. A lot of times students and residents think they have to do what they're told and can't contribute to the pharmacy," she explained.

"I know, I guess I'm used to my father and just doing what I'm told. I want to contribute, but I don't want to step on any toes," I offered, noticing my anger start to brim.

She calibrated her tone to match mine. "You aren't just a peon. You and I are on the same level."

Memories were triggered from Winn Drugs. *You are just an intern. I'm the pharmacist.* I was pissed. Overwhelmed. INFURIATED.

I got up and tried to gather my pocketbook and coat to leave.

"CHRISTINA. WAIT," she boomed. "What is causing this strong reaction from you?"

"You said I was a peon. I don't need to be spoken to like this! I'm leaving!" I yelled, tears forming in my eyes.

"I didn't mean you were a peon. I was saying you and I are equals and I want to hear your opinion," she responded firmly, but patiently.

I wanted to escape. To go smoke a cigarette or eat or take a shot of vodka. But something held me in the office that day. My pride was out the window but something deep inside me desperately wanted to heal. Somewhere inside, behind the pain and hurt, was a strong-ass desire to heal.

"Christina, sit down. Let's talk about this."

I obliged, surprising myself.

"You are being triggered by your past. I understand that. I went through similar things with my family. I want you to know I never want to hurt you and I am here to help you grow."

I collapsed into her arms and cried. "I'm sorry. I feel lonely and I'm in so much mental pain. I can't ignore it," I said through broken sobs. It was a defining moment. This was surely my rock bottom, sitting in an office crying in my residency director's arms.

The beautiful thing about rock bottom is that you can only go up from that point. I knew things needed to change. And like many of my other searches, it started on Google.

Later that day, I typed the three words into the search tab: "Eating disorder therapists."

Columbia center for eating disorders, Psychology Today listing of ED specialists, the eating disorder resource center. A random ED Meetup in NYC. Sounded good; it was free. They met one Saturday a month. The group leader's name was Judie Stein. Her picture appeared in the top-left corner of the page. She had highlighted medium-length blonde hair, a genuine smile and kind-looking face. I had met several therapists in the past and most of them were rigid and just wanted to "treat" you. Something about her authenticity made me want to read on....

I am a therapist, divorce mediator, and adjunct professor at NYU with a specialization in eating disorders. I am interested in helping to facilitate a monthly meet-up group to discuss experiences, treatment options, and helpful ideas in dealing with eating disorders of all types. I have years of experience treating bulimia, binge eating, anorexia, and issues of body image, with excellent results.

In addition to seeing patients individually for eating disorders (among other issues), I'm currently forming an ongoing, weekly therapy group for persons with eating disorders who are looking for something more ongoing and intensive. I work on a sliding fee scale, so I will do what I can to make it work for you. My approach is a combination of psychodynamic, cognitive-behavioral, and Buddhist principles, with a healthy dose of compassion and understanding!

Our meet ups are held in Union Square, near 12th Street and University Place.

Please give me a call or email me if you think you might be interested in attending the meet-ups or in learning more about individual or group therapy. Space is somewhat limited, so if you are interested, it's best to call or email me right away.

Thank you!
Judie Stein, Ph.D., L.M.S.W.

I was torn. A part of me wanted to go, but another part said it wasn't that bad. It wasn't like I was a drug user or an alcoholic. I just ate at night to numb my feelings. That wasn't too abnormal, right? I clicked "Yes" for the RSVP and closed the tab on my computer as Dr. Chawla walked into the office, and I went back to work.

I didn't yet know how much that "Yes" would alter my life. It was one of the biggest steps I had ever taken toward true healing.

People will spend days, weeks, months, and years in mental and physical pain. They will stay wrapped in an argument and remain firm in their convictions because they have to be right. I spent two years battling forgiveness and processing what had happened to me. I was like a tiger trapped in a cage, ravenous for more fuel to prove I had been the victim. The ego is a nasty animal and will judge, blame, and create separation amongst people. Yet the ego will fight you tooth and nail to keep you in that addiction, in that abusive relationship or unfulfilling job. Your *soul* always knows the way to healing and the way to get there.

Living in accordance to your ego has a cost. My ego kept me in an unfulfilling job for 7 years. It cost me several essential pieces of my happiness.

Playing small and giving my power and energy away cost me my:

Health: I was waking up every night eating junk food, over-exercising and addicted to sugar.

Freedom: I felt as if I had something to prove, a way to say "screw you" to my parents.

Creativity: My energy was invested in the drama and pain and left little for work. I was constantly drinking coffee and eating sugar to keep my energy up.

Joy: I was isolating myself because I wanted to be successful and became a workaholic. Personal relationships were not high on my priority list—including loving relationships with my family and myself.

True fulfillment: My *soul* kept nudging me toward healing, but my ego would draw me back.

In order to begin the journey to revealing your true self, you have to begin to *listen* to yourself. Sometimes people will not begin to listen until they hit rock bottom. They may half listen and try to break free, but until you listen fully and *surrender* to something higher than yourself, you stay stuck.

Rock bottom may occur as different events for people. A divorce. A hard breakup. A death. A life-threatening illness. It may take something that rips your heart out, breaks you open and never leaves you the same again. This is your awakening. It's a wake-up call for you to take a serious inventory of what you've been denying about yourself, take your power back, and surrender to the deeper lesson. What you don't realize is that your breakdowns can actually propel you toward your biggest breakthroughs.

This awakening is meant to crack you wide open so you can shed those limiting beliefs of who you thought you were. You see, we are all born with unique gifts and talents that were meant to be utilized to help the greater good in this world. Your creator embedded those gifts in your heart at birth to be expressed to amplify love and help mankind. As we grow as children, often our parents want to protect or control us and unintentionally block those natural gifts. In another case, maybe kids at school ridicule a child so the child hides their true ability. We are shaped by our environment and we fear being rejected, which are two big reasons we may have stifled or ignored our own precious gifts and talents — and if our gifts and talents are not nurtured and appreciated in childhood, we find it difficult or even impossible to express them as adults. When this happens, we tend to feel empty and unfulfilled.

The same is true for how children develop and come to identify with who they are. Children naturally model the beliefs and ideas of the family of origin, or their parents. Feelings of unworthiness, of not being good enough, or any other limiting beliefs are often implanted in us before the age of 6. As we grow into teenagers and adults, these limiting beliefs constrict us mentally and emotionally, limiting what we will reach for in life. Limiting beliefs hold people back in every aspect of life — financially, emotionally, mentally and physically. The truth is, we are *unlimited* in what we can do and achieve. If you want to change a behavior, you need to start by changing your beliefs.

I needed some serious belief adjustments during that time of my life. When I was at that lowest part in my life, I was isolated from my family, depressed, anxious, and lonely. But I never gave up. I believed I would find the resources and support to heal even if my family didn't support me. The healing for my eating disorder started with Judie Stein.

Chapter 21: Don't you...forget about me

Judie Stein was a petite Jewish woman with a bright smile and a kind heart. I know because I felt her energy emanating with compassion at every interaction. After years of practice with Adrienne, I was now used to talk-therapy. Judie helped me to further see my distortions as I discovered just *how* hard I was on myself. I began to cultivate love and compassion for the parts of myself that I had once hated.

Each week we would talk about what emotional triggers were coming up for me, how I was doing with my eating at night, and how my relationships were going. I didn't know how to connect with myself other than with food. It wasn't an intelligence thing—I understood what was healthy, how much I should be exercising, etc. There is an implicit interplay between attempting to control life through food. It was an *emotional* thing. And I was very emotional.

I spoke to Judie about my deepest fears, of being judged by my parents and never being good enough or worthy enough to be loved. I knew I had to reconcile with my parents somehow. Judie helped me realize that I had to find the right tools to work through my problems. You can't build a house with a hammer and a saw. You need nails, cement, wood—all of those materials and tools to build a strong foundation first.

I had all of the wrong tools—no support, isolation, binge eating, and drinking alcohol. Plus I was bitter, angry, and resentful. I was hard on myself and others and had constant mood swings from sugar/caffeine addiction. I was extremely frustrated with my life situation.

Slowly but surely, I began softening my heart for my father. *His* wounding was a projection of his own fears and demons. I was simply on the receiving end. It was a growing experience for me to leave the house, start an independent life, and find my true self. I needed to separate from my parents to get out of that environment.

I was feeling more confident about myself as I was beginning to unmask my pain to reveal the layers of who I really was at the core. I came to know FEARS as Fuck Everything and Run Strategies. They were all bullshit!

For 2013, I mapped out a plan of action—setting spiritual, mental/relationship, and physical goals for myself. I promised not to ever betray my own heart, and to honor, love, and respect myself. I praised myself for sticking to my plan when I could have given up on my dream and crawled back to my parents. There were many points that I didn't know how I would get through the pain because it was so deep. Yet I kept moving forward. I had to.

One day at the pharmacy I was in such a great mood, bursting with my newfound self-love. I had listened to house music on the way to work. However that day Dr. Chawla's energy completely threw me off—it was draining and low. It was then that I realized how susceptible I was to people's energy fields. I literally took on the emotions of others. My upper back would tense up like a cat with the fur on edge. I asked her what was wrong and she said something about her son being sick and coming home from daycare. I saw the tears in her eyes and felt her pain. I lit the lavender candle in our office and gave her a hug.

Dr. Chawla knew every bit of what I was going through. She and I exchanged dozens of conversations about fear, growth, rejection, and pain. One day, I unlocked my door and turned on the lights to find a tiny elephant on my desk.

"What is this? Is this a present for me?" I asked Dr. Chawla.

"I know you're going through a tough time with your family. His name is Ganesha, a Hindu diety. He's known as the Remover of Obstacles," she explained.

"Thank you," I said, my heart opening for the first time in a long time. "This means so much to me!"

Ganesha—the elephant-deity riding a mouse—has become one of the most common mnemonics for anything associated with Hinduism. He has an elephantine countenance with a curved trunk and big ears, and a huge pot-bellied body of a human being. Ganesha is the lord of success and destroyer of evils and obstacles. He is also worshipped as the god of education, knowledge, wisdom, and wealth. Ganesha's head symbolizes the *Atman* or the soul, which is the ultimate supreme reality of human existence, and his human body signifies *Maya* or the earthly existence of human beings. I was so grateful for this elephant—the remover of obstacles. I was grateful for life.

And then a series of synchronistic events happened that changed everything.

Chapter 22: Ohhhh sometimes I get a good feeling, a little feeling that I never knew before…

One day on my lunch break, I headed to a local juice bar to order a wheatgrass shot. It was my daily dose of "health" to convince myself I was still healthy, even though I ate so horribly at night. I looked up at the dark Ecuadorian man who was making the wheatgrass shot. When he handed it across the counter, I cringed.

"Can I have a chaser, please? I hate this taste. Wheatgrass is such a superfood" — I rambled off the wealth of amino acids, nutrients, and minerals it contains — "but it tastes like garbage."

He smiled, pouring me a small cup of OJ. "Ah, I know the taste is not so pleasant. But yes! Wheatgrass is full of amino acids and so many minerals that benefit the skin and all of the organs. I love nutrition — I actually went to Integrative Nutrition and learned a lot about health and wellness."

I nodded, then knocked back the wheatgrass shot and chaser.

"If you like nutrition, you should sign up for the course and become a health coach," he added.

My eyes widened as I gulped it down. I had never heard of a health coach before, but I was intrigued. I knew it was a sign from the universe to jump for this opportunity. I called the school that day only to find that the tuition cost $4,000. *Shit. Roadblock.* I told the representative I would call back.

It cost $4,000 for a 12-month course to become a health coach. After 6 months in the program, you could take on clients as a consultant and enroll them into your 6-month wellness program. I was a resident making $17 an hour. How could I afford this kind of investment?

My internal conflict must have shown on my face because Dr. Chawla knew something wasn't right that day and asked me what was wrong.

"I have such a bad poker face. I wear my heart on my sleeve…. It costs a lot of money for Integrative Nutrition," I told her solemnly.

"Yes, but it's an investment in your future. You have to know your worth and be willing to invest in yourself. If money wasn't an object, how excited would you be to start the program?"

"Oh, I am so enthusiastic about it. If money wasn't an object, I would sign up right away."

"Well think back to how you decided you wanted to become a pharmacist. You can draw upon your past decisions and look at your thought process to make sure you're making the right choice now."

"I just remember watching my father at his pharmacy and I had this feeling in my chest…this expansive feeling, almost like I'd experienced love for the first time. I saw him genuinely serving and it sparked something inside me that wouldn't let me turn away. Since then, I've always wanted to help and serve others..." I explained.

"Christina...did you just hear what you said? You became a pharmacist because of a *feeling*, because you wanted to capture a moment in time. And while a pharmacist does spend time counseling patients, a retail pharmacist does the bulk of their work behind the counter, on the phone, typing prescriptions, etc." She was right.

"I know. That's why I wanted to do a residency and see what else was out there. I wanted to learn how to implement and foster my own programs and administer vaccines, compound medications—all of that. I want to be challenged. And now I want to deepen the relationships with my patients through this health coaching. So I need to do it," I declared.

"Then I would really think about what you just said. If you feel in alignment, do it! Before you make a decision, meditate on it. Do hot yoga. Get into the space of alignment."

"Alignment" had become a part of our daily vernacular, as did words like "connected" and "the journey." As you are aligning with your true desires, you are aligning with your higher self. To be in alignment means to hold a thought and/or belief which feels emotionally positive and therefore resonates at the same frequency as your desire. This is your indication that you're in line with your higher self, and subsequently, that the manifestation of your desire (into the physical dimension) will occur.

Dr. Chawla went to grab coffee and I thought deeply about our conversation. I had been chasing a feeling for 10 years…since I was 14 years old. It only took one split second for me to decide on my career path. At the time, it felt like such a huge pull on my heart, like an external force steering me, with the bells and whistles and billboard signs saying "HEY THIS IS YOUR LIFE'S PURPOSE! DON'T YOU DARE TURN AWAY!" Now I wasn't so sure if pharmacy was my true calling. What else would I do? What was my *purpose* here?

"I've been chasing a feeling for 10 years," I wrote on an orange sticky note and stuck it on Dr. Chawla's desk before leaving to go do TPNs.

As I was preparing my daily compounds in the compounding room, I drifted into thought…. Dr. Chawla and I were both on a path of self-discovery, of reinventing ourselves, of staying in the space of deep connection to God and our purpose. Since I was 18 I had this tug on my heart to become more, to give more in this world. I began questioning everything I had known and these questions led me to write daily, to want to connect with nature at the Long Beach boardwalk, to continue on the path in pharmacy to serve others. I had an intuition to one day write a book to touch thousands of people. I envisioned my story reaching all of those lost souls in the world who had disordered eating. In my mind, no one should suffer and be left without support like I had been. There was always a solution. As Dr. Chawla taught me, "You need tools and support when going through a transformation." And I sure as hell was transforming.

After compounding, I returned to an empty office. It was 5:30 and everyone had filtered out of the office. The orange Post-it rested on my desk. Curiously, I picked it up and realized Dr. Chawla had written underneath what I wrote....

"Wouldn't you rather chase your feeling rather than someone else's dream?"

A huge smile spread across my face. This was the one Post-it I would keep for a very long time.

Yes. Of course. That was the very reason why I was going to invest $4,000, kiss it up to God, trust the universe, and sign up for Integrative Nutrition.

I wasn't exactly sure how I would do the residency full-time and go through the Integrative Nutrition program, but I had faith and a burning desire to impact my future clients. Plus I was Joe Tarantola's daughter—an overachiever with a burning desire to make the world better.

A week later, I received a huge red package from Integrative Nutrition filled with marketing materials, the Fast Track handbook, and the Integrative Nutrition book. That night I peeled open the IIN to the Table of Contents and was drawn to the Deconstructing Cravings chapter. Joshua Rosenthal was both the founder of IIN and the author of the book I was holding. He was an amicable, bald hippie who wanted nothing more than peace and love for the world. I'd heard him talk in my audio lectures and loved how authentic and genuine his message was. I started reading the chapter and fell into the pages, engulfed by his rationale behind what caused food cravings. He was basically saying that our bodies know how to heal themselves and our bodies always want to return to homeostasis—balance and stability.

If something is wrong within us, in order to restore balance our brain triggers our body to crave certain foods. Often what we crave is connection and love, but instead we fill that emptiness with food. I learned that people often medicate themselves with food, and I was no exception.

I devoured the material, feeling as if IIN was divinely guiding me. I had been so concerned with helping others when I really needed help myself, and I had lost myself in the process. It was what I had done my whole life—please and assist others. IIN was a program to help me teach others how to live a full, healthy, abundant life, but I had to heal first. It was *my* time.

Part II

Chapter 23: And constant craving has always been...

As I was going through IIN, I was also learning to teach diabetes classes under the direction of Dr. Chawla. When people are first diagnosed with a disease, they deal with a range of emotions— denial, grief, guilt, shame, anger, or all of these. Each person has a unique experience of their illness and what brings them to a diabetes class. As a guide for them, I was both an educator and a support system, providing a safe space for their worries and concerns to be heard with dignity and respect. It was a healing space, and many of the patients connected with each other as they related through their similar experiences.

During that time, I began researching more about how food could help heal disease and I became particularly interested in functional medicine. I studied the pH diet, the plant-based diet, the vegetarian diet, and the anti-inflammatory diet. I traveled to Asheville, North Carolina for an Alternative Medicine Symposium to hear Dr. Andrew Weil speak. He taught his patients the 4-7-8 breathing technique, which helps stress reduction. He also talked about the anti-inflammatory diet and mindfulness practices, which could help chronic diseases like Irritable Bowel Syndrome.

I began to incorporate all of this information into my diabetes classes, educating my patients about how adding more green leafy vegetables can lower Hemoglobin A1C, the average measurement of a person's blood sugar over a 3-month period. I taught them about how diabetes affected their body, long-term health, and how to prevent complications like amputation, blindness, and kidney disease.

"Picture a full glass of water. Now picture dumping a huge amount of sugar into it. That is what happens with diabetes. What would the consistency be like?" I would probe the patients to make them understand how diabetes affected their blood. "If your bloodstream has too much sugar in it and is too thick, the blood can't get to your brain or your heart or any other organ. This puts you at an increased risk of a stroke, heart attack, or kidney disease," I told them.

This information sparked individual conversations within the class that opened up questions for my patients to understand how nutrition impacted their disease.

One day, as I was teaching a class on food cravings, a patient interjected with an interesting comment.

"I really have a sweet tooth and can't control my cravings — what does that mean?" she asked.

"Well, sweet cravings can come from so many things. It's our bodies craving for comfort, safety, and security. We want connection and most of the time food produces a certainty that we can have connection. When we want macaroni and cheese or a cookie, it's comforting. Sometimes we're just tired and a simple carbohydrate gives us a rush of energy. Other times we're bored and eat a bowl of ice cream because it feels good."

What I was trying to explain to her is the phenomenon that is so deeply ingrained in our human wiring. Hunger signals can be so powerful, yet so deceiving. Sometimes the mind takes over and makes us think we're hungry, when we're really craving connection, touch, or even love. Food is so deeply connected to social gatherings, holidays, even going on dates to the movies. A rich bar of chocolate and soda sends strong pleasure signals to the brain and provides comfort. On the flip side, in order to avoid feeling, a compulsive eater may use food to numb and suppress harsh emotions. Shame, anger, guilt, and self-hatred are just some of those dense emotions that can trigger a binge episode. Using food to numb emotions leaves the person in a cycle of guilt.

I saw the world through a new lens and started attracting people who needed the advice I had learned. One of my first clients, Helen, was told from childhood that she was fat and "big-boned." She didn't trust men and thought they only wanted to use her for sex. At the core of her hopelessness and depression was a deep self-hatred and she would take trips to fast food restaurants then vomit all of the food up. She was never "full," and the memories of her parents' harsh words haunted her. I supported her by reading her food logs and helping her to understand where her cravings came from. She began examining her limiting beliefs in therapy and joined an Overeaters Anonymous group for additional support. As her shame of never being good enough lifted, so did her pounds of pain. The process of her healing was incredible and inspired me to continue on my path to help others heal.

The same process happened for me. I was ashamed of my choice to be a health coach and a healer and to leave my father's pharmacy. For so long I had been a people-pleaser, pushing my own needs aside. I wasn't connected to myself and I felt completely empty inside.

During that time I was healing and soaking up new knowledge, the picture of disease became very real to me. Disease stood front and center as I learned that my father was diagnosed with Congestive Heart Failure. Over time, he had been complaining of extreme fatigue that he attributed to just "getting older." After several heart tests, the doctor confirmed that my father had to change his lifestyle in order to live.

One day I walked into the house around Christmas time. My mother was adorning the tree with our vibrant Christopher Radko ornaments. I always loved that cozy feeling of coming home to a house filled with Christmas decorations. My father walked into the living room to meet us near the tree.

"Hey Dad. I heard what happened at the doctor's the other day," I said, hugging him without care if he would give me a reciprocal strong hug. I pulled away from his body, feeling a catch in my chest like someone just hit me with a baseball in the sternum. The tears came.

"Yeah. I'm fine, though," he said. Stoic. Strong. Enduring. "Want to see my medicine?" he asked like a small child showing me his new Tonka trucks.

"Sure, Dad."

I walked into his bathroom with the old white plastic cabinets that sprang open from the loose glue on the seam. He opened the loose cabinet and took out a blue plastic pill box.

"See, I have to take about 5 pills a day. No big deal." He shrugged it off, popping a tiny Carvedilol pill into his mouth.

I took the weight for both of us and continued crying. *We have helped other people who were sick. I stood side by side with him for years counting pills like these. It isn't right to see him taking these.*

"Christina...don't cry. I'm fine. I'm going to live!" he said, trying to cheer me up. I couldn't help but feel guilty for this in some way. *Did I break his heart? Did I induce this heart failure?* Some of those thoughts roamed my brain for days and stayed. Other thoughts left over time. *I have to heal this somehow.*

In therapy, I came to release the anger from my early childhood years and separate what had happened to who I was as an adult. When a traumatic event occurs, we adapt a certain behavior or coping mechanism such as withdrawal, aggression, crying, etc. That coping mechanism served us as children because we had to "survive." As adults, this maladaptive behavior impacts us on a daily basis. In order to heal and move on from the original event, you have to be willing to examine, release, and accept the past.

Prescription for Connecting with Your Soul Desire/Life Purpose:

So I ask you, what is it you *really* want? What is your soul calling for? Love? Self-love? Spirituality? Fulfillment through your life purpose? Connecting meaningfully with people you love? I promise you, the answer is not in your refrigerator, in others approval, or in alcohol or drugs. It is within you and all you have to do is be still enough to listen. You have all the answers inside you already.

To connect with your soul's desire, try this visualization exercise:

1. Sit quietly for 2 minutes. Think of a time when you were most happy in life. What were you doing? Where were you? Who was with you? What smells, sounds, and pictures come to mind?

2. Take in the scene and stay connected to it. Feel how you felt that day. Were you in love with someone at the time? Were you connecting with strangers on a road trip? Were you having your first child? What memory conjures up the strongest positive memory for you?

3. Pay attention to this memory. Follow your bliss and your passions — always. What you are passionate about is most likely what you are meant for.

I used to have visions of speaking in front of thousands of people and being a published author. It was God's way of showing me what I was called here to do. Practice this meditation daily. This is what meditation might be like for you, simply being a witness to your thoughts.

Write your thoughts and insights here:

_____

_____

_____

_____

_____

Chapter 24: Cause it's the eye of the tiger, it's the thrill of the fight, risin' up to the challenge of our rivals

Despite these blessings that were manifesting for me, I still wasn't feeling like myself. I had not gone to the gym in months because I rationalized that I didn't want to waste money on it. I had bills and was getting paid very little at my job.

My angel, Dr. Chawla, stepped in to show me another lesson.

"I used to love going to the gym," I explained to her. "I don't want to go to the gym in Howard Beach, and Crunch across the street is expensive. I just really miss working out and getting the 'high' after."

"Well, why don't you go check out the rates across the street? Remember to self-care you have to be willing to invest in yourself. You are worth it," she reminded me.

Quite frankly, I didn't want to spend that kind of money on myself. I had been taught to work hard and save. I didn't understand where these ideas of "not having enough" were coming from. Then it came to me: a memory of my father commenting on how egg whites cost an extra $1.00 on a breakfast sandwich. *Really, Dad?*

Investing in myself to get a massage, a facial, or any amount of self-care felt selfish and wasteful to me. The money I spent on therapy, rent, and other bills was killing me as it was. I could buy several meals with that money. I could pay my electric bill. I wasn't used to investing in myself for my mental, emotional, or spiritual growth. An underlying worthlessness existed within me. *How can I break that pattern? Take small steps, Christina,* was how my consciousness answered the question.

I decided my mentor was right and hopped across the street one day after work to Crunch. It was a beautiful gym with cardio machines upstairs and downstairs, saunas, spin classes, weights, you name it. It was $80 a month…. Again I had a decision to make. I made a meager salary and had bills to pay every month. Was it worth it to pay another $80 a month? Did I want to be happy? Did I think I deserved to be happy? Yes. I needed to lift weights and attend classes to feel like myself again. I forked over my MasterCard and cringed as it was swiped. *I trust myself. I love myself.*

I started going to Crunch 3 to 4 times a week and the trainers in the gym were extremely helpful. They would reposition my arms while I was lifting weights to help me target the right muscle groups. One trainer in particular, Eugene, had so much energy. He would walk around the gym with his chest puffed out and give random gym members high-fives.

"Yeah! Getting to the DAMN goals!" he would shout as everyone else turned their heads with a bewildered look. I laughed but secretly his energy raised mine. I felt motivated after hearing him shout. I had never seen someone with such enthusiasm. He stopped to talk to me about training one day and I couldn't help but ask him what his secret was for being so outwardly excited about life. I wanted his happiness elixir.

"Have you ever heard of Tony Robbins?" he asked.

"No, who is that?"

"Oh my goodness. You don't know TONY ROBBINS?! He's a motivational speaker, he's written books and holds seminars about personal development. I went to his Unleash the Power Within event in LA and it changed my life. You need to read his books," he said, beaming. I admired the confidence and authority in his voice.

"Okay, I'll have to go buy one of his books. Which one should I start with?"

"*Awaken the Giant Within* is a great one to start. He talks about eliminating limiting beliefs that hold you back from reaching your full potential. You'll love it." He grinned.

Anthony Robbins helped people "raise the standards" in their life. In other words, take no shit and get your act together. I was tired of being tired, and I was thirsty for answers. I went to Barnes and Noble to buy the Tony Robbins book. It was a thick 500 pages and I swept it right off the shelf, eager to go home to my apartment and read it.

I drove back to Howard Beach around 1pm, prepared to lose power that night. It was the day right before Hurricane Sandy swept through the Northeast. I was in Zone A. I closed my blinds as the winds started picking up and the tiny tree outside my first-floor window undulated in the gust. I was too afraid to leave the blinds open. *What if the water came all the way to Lindenwood?* I pushed that thought out of my mind and focused on the book. As I was placing triple-A batteries in the reading light, I started thinking about my own internal storm. How could this situation ever be solved? Was there a way to restore my relationship with my family? My gut told me probably not, that my father would hold this grudge for a very long time. *No negative thoughts, Christina.* I opened the book to the first page.

> *We all have dreams.... We all want to believe deep down in our souls that we have a special gift, that we can make a difference, that we can touch others in a special way, and that we can make the world a better place. At a very early age I developed a belief that we're all here to contribute something unique, that deep within each of us lies a special gift. You see, I truly believe we all have a sleeping giant within us. Each of us has a talent, a gift, our own bit of genius just waiting to be tapped. I've learned that the resources we need to turn our dreams into reality are within us, merely waiting for the day when we decide to wake up and claim our birthright. I wrote this book for one reason: to be a wake-up call that will challenge those who are committed to living and being more to take their God-given power.*

> *You see, I believe I know who you really are. I believe you and I must be kindred souls. Your desire to expand has brought you to this book. Deep inside of you there lies a belief that your experience of life can and will be much greater than it already is. You are destined for your own unique form of greatness, whether it is as an outstanding professional, teacher, businessperson, mother or father. By consistently taking advantage of each of the chapters in this book, you'll ensure your ability to maximize your potential. I challenge you not only to do whatever it takes to read this book in its entirety, but also to use what you learn in simple ways each day.*

I was hooked. It felt like he was a friend talking to me personally in the form of writing. Yes, I had always known I had a purpose, a message to spread! Yes, I am committed to living a bigger life! How do I fulfill my potential? Reach thousands of people? Make changes to be as effective as possible?

That day, in my studio apartment, I became absolutely enamored by the message in this book. I hung on Tony Robbins' every word, marveling at his resilience to overcome thick barriers just like I had. He had gotten kicked out of his house, gained 38 pounds and had lived in a tiny studio apartment. He'd made a list of things he would no longer tolerate in his life and everything he aspired to become. He gave a step-by-step approach to changing maladaptive patterns. He spoke about raising your standards. He would no longer settle for a life less than extraordinary.

A huge part of his teaching was about changing limiting beliefs, the ideas and thoughts you've told yourself for years but that don't serve you. It's the voice that tells you what is and isn't possible. In order to reach your maximum potential, Robbins explained, you have to become aware of what story you're telling yourself about your past and dissemble it to reach greatness. You see, people cling to the past and become victims to their "story." Everyone has a story, and attaching meaning to the story creates suffering. Our subconscious recognizes patterns from our past and causes us to react in certain ways to protect ourselves from pain. We are creatures of condition, much like Pavlov's dogs.

I got out my journal and started doing the exercises outlined in the book. I wrote down my empowering and disempowering beliefs:

Empowering beliefs
If I am myself, I will attract love and the right partner.
If I honor my values and goals, my dreams will come true.
If I stay in pharmacy, I want to focus on consulting.

Limiting beliefs:
If I don't do what people want, they will retract money and love from me.
I am not worthy of being happy.
I am bad for leaving my family.

Disempowering beliefs
The hurt and pain from being rejected by my family is a heavy feeling for me.
It is tough to trust people in this world. Many people do things only because they want something in return.

I finished the lengthy book in 2 days during Hurricane Sandy, scribbling in the margins and completing the exercises in my journal. Tony Robbins became my coach, mentor, teacher and inspiration. I would watch his YouTube videos on my laptop since I had no television and revel in how compelling his energy was. I bought his CDs and would listen to them on my way to work. He said that in order to be a leader you had to commit to emotional, physical, relationship, financial, and time mastery.

His message showed me that the key to real change was to make a decision to say "NO MORE." I knew I wanted to make an impact in the lives of thousands of people and I never wanted people to feel the way I did—lost, confused, heavy, depressed. I made it my mission to raise my standards and heal myself. In turn, I promised myself that once I was healed, I would do anything in my power to help others.

In order to begin to change, there has to be a *willingness* to do so. I can always tell when someone is "checked out" or avoiding keeping appointments with me that they are not ready to really change. The TransTheoretical Model (TTM) of Change states that there are 5 stages of change. The 6th one, relapse, is optional and does not happen for everyone. This idea of motivational interviewing originated when psychologists were trying to help people out of alcohol and drug addictions, however it can be used to change any behavior, such as to quit smoking or recover from an eating disorder. Motivational interviewing uses this algorithm along with different counseling tools to guide people to break habits.

The 5 Stages are:

1. Pre-contemplation phase – Person has no intention to change and is reluctant to admit they have a problem. They may rationalize why the behavior is okay to continue.

2. Contemplation phase – In this stage the person is willing to consider treatment and acknowledge that they have a problem. However they are still on the fence about starting treatment.

3.   Preparation phase – The decision is made to stop the behavior. Commitment and determination to change requires a realistic plan and support. People will usually take action in the next month. A motivating belief usually propels people to enter into the next phase.

4.   Action phase – Individuals at this stage will enter treatment or seek counseling. They seek an external support network to keep them accountable and cheer them on.

5.   Maintenance phase – This phase takes 3 to 6 months. The threat of old patterns becomes null or insignificant and confidence increases.

6.   Relapse – There is always a possibility for relapse, but keeping a strong positive support network is key to prevent and deal with relapse.

When a coach or therapist is assessing which stage a client or patient is at, they will use certain language to help explore the underlying motives. It's important to get to the *why*—or the motivating factor underlying the need to change a behavior. My big *why* to change was to feel more energized and fulfill my life purpose to inspire people through my writing. What is your motivation to change?

Prescription for Empowerment:

1.   What are your limiting beliefs about why you are not happy right now?

_____

_____

_____

_____

2.   What   are   your   disempowering/empowering
beliefs about your health? Your finances? Your relationship?

_____

_____

_____

_____

3.   What stage of change are you at in being ready to
change a current behavior? Whether it's smoking, alcohol,
food addiction, or another destructive pattern.

_____

_____

_____

_____

4.   What action steps can you take today to change
that behavior? Ask for support by talking to a coach,
therapist, church leader or objective friend. What tools and
resources can you tap into to learn more about the
condition?

_____

_____

_____

_____

Chapter 25: So raise your glass if you are wrong in all the right ways

There are endless opportunities to nourish your body throughout the day. There are so many nutritional supplements available now that it can be overwhelming. You can choose to take vitamins, minerals and wheatgrass shots, and drink green juices or nutritional shakes. Many nutritional companies promote their brand as the best to shed weight, burn fat, and increase energy—so which one do you choose? Do you simply eat a well-balanced diet that incorporates those vitamins and minerals?

As individuals, each of us has a unique biochemistry and genetic makeup. This is called our *bioindividuality*. What may work for you may not work for another person.

I remember teaching my diabetes classes and having one of the patients read her blood sugar log to the class.

"I ate a bowl of instant oatmeal at 8:30am and an hour later my blood sugar shot up 100 points! I can't eat oatmeal anymore."

Another patient said, "I was fine with that same oatmeal. I eat oatmeal every day and my blood sugar stays stable."

I explained to the group that each person's body responds to food in a unique way. Some people are more sensitive to carbohydrates than others. This is why some people with diabetes have higher insulin requirements. You can't compare apples to oranges. You have to tune into your own body to understand what works best for you.

That being said, there are two things we have in life at any moment: choice and awareness. Many people, including myself, have chosen to eat foods that do not nourish their body. Let me preface this with, yes, you *will* eat an occasional cheeseburger, slice of New York-style pizza, or a piece of cheesecake. No diet or way of eating will ever be picture-perfect. That is normal and healthy! What I'm saying is that continual overconsumption of foods that lack nutrients will ultimately contribute and lead to food addiction and disease in the body.

Many people are addicted to food and may not be aware that they are numbing their emotions by *using* food. I shy away from such terms as "emotional eaters" to avoid labeling anyone as having a 'disease' or disorder. You are much more than a label or a behavior. You are a beautiful, feeling human being. However, many people eat when they are emotional. Stress, anger, frustration, guilt, and many other emotions can trigger a binge. The way to become more aware of this pattern is to not dissociate from your feelings.

Dissociating from your emotions happens when you "step outside of yourself" and disconnect from yourself. It is too painful to feel those feelings so you dissociate. Trauma typically precedes dissociation and can stem from psychological, sexual, or physical abuse.

What is a "trauma?" If some event in your life produced an intense emotional response, it is a trauma. Do not minimize what happened to you, even if it's small compared to other people. I have heard many people say, "Well, I have no right to complain about my father ignoring me or verbally abusing me. There are people out there who have been sexually abused." If it's relevant and significant to you, then it was traumatic.

When I had my eating disorder, I used food as my crutch. I would deprive myself of nutrients during the day and stay rigid in how I ate, portioning everything out perfectly. Then when I came home at night, I would binge on cookies and cereal in shame. It was all or nothing. There was no middle ground where I would allow myself to be in touch with what I really wanted or needed.

So much of food addiction is tied to emotional eating. I used food to numb heavy emotions like loneliness, pain, and anger, and to fill the emptiness I felt. Often, binge eating quells those feelings because of a chemical response from the brain as well as the temporary feeling of fullness that follows.

Self-medication with food to ease tension, depression, or anxiety is common, and most people with this pattern have similar sensations that are likened to drug withdrawal. When you take away the substance, the body feels the effects, just like a drug. You may feel headache, nausea, and strong mood changes. Racing thoughts trigger emotions, which trigger overeating. Lessening the heavy emotions and learning to cope is how you begin to overcome emotional eating.

How do you know you're addicted to food?
1. Compulsive use of the substance despite negative health and social consequences

2.   Tolerance – over time, progressively greater amounts of the substance are needed to reach and maintain the "high"

3.   Withdrawal symptoms (toxic hunger) when the substance is discontinued

4.   Activation of reward pathways (including the dopamine system) in the brain and the impulsive need to consume

The origin of food addiction is inherent in our food supply. Americans have the most overweight citizens in the world. I cannot help but think that a contributory factor is because of the hydrogenated oil, high fructose corn syrup, and chemicals in the bulk of what we consume. Many are not *aware* that McDonald's and other fast-food chains submerge their fries and burgers in food additives that increase a person's craving for the food. Many foods and beverages such as soda, breads, ketchup, and cereals have high fructose corn syrup, which alters satiety hormones that tell your brain when you're full. These chemicals increase appetite and lead to weight gain and insulin resistance.

The power of choice and what food/beverages we put into our bodies is dependent on so many things — taste, convenience, and a physiological response to food additives that increase cravings for certain foods.

Researchers have done MRIs on the human brain after the subject ate a candy bar and the same area of the brain lit up as that of a person who was on cocaine. Eating a sweet piece of chocolate triggers intense feelings and memories about pleasure as well as activating dopamine receptors in the brain. These feelings originate from the dopamine reward system. (Dopamine is a neurochemical that regulates motivation, pleasure, and reinforcement related to certain stimuli—such as food.) The amount of pleasure we derive from eating a food correlates with the amount of dopamine released in the brain.

Also, neuroimaging has been done to prove that obese individuals have a less sensitive response to dopamine due to a down regulation of receptors in the brain. This means there are less receptor sites for dopamine, which is why an obese individual needs more of the substance (food) to achieve the effect (pleasure). It will take an obese person a higher quantity of food to feel the effects of fullness and pleasure. They have a greater desire for food with a diminished reward response. This is why many people have sugar cravings that cannot be quelled by a single handful of M&Ms.

I have found several powerful tools to increase awareness and create leverage to choose healthy foods. Some are related directly to food and others are mental/emotional/spiritual tools. I will discuss all of these so you feel empowered to take control of your life again. You may feel hopeless when you are constantly in a cycle of food addiction or numbing your feelings. I promise you, there is a way out.

The first tool you can utilize is to keep a food log of how you feel with each food you eat immediately after you eat it, then one hour after. Write down how your body feels, your level of energy from 0 to 10, and how your mood is affected. Certain people are intolerant to gluten, dairy, or caffeine. You may have been so busy throughout your day that you did not even pay attention to how food affected your energy and mood.

Logging your food and writing down how you feel afterward will serve two purposes. First, you will become mindful of everything you are eating and drinking. Doing this may surprise you! You may notice you are continuously noshing throughout the day, grabbing a handful of your kids' fries or drinking more soda than you thought. The second function it serves is connecting what you eat to how your body feels. This is different than how your mind perceives the food. If you connect what you eat with how you feel, you will naturally want to choose more healthful foods.

Remember the story I told about the woman whose blood sugar shot up 100 points after consuming that hearty bowl of oats? This will be a key to open the door to how *your* body operates. Everyone is so different and is on a unique path to their health and healing journey. Once you know what works and doesn't work for you, eating well will become so much easier.

This is how I began healing my eating disorder. As I was teaching my patients about healthy eating and balancing blood sugar to prevent weight gain, I became aware that I was *not* taking care of myself. I would eat a processed breakfast sandwich, a small piece of chicken with vegetables for lunch, and then come home and eat a small dinner. Then at night I would wake up to eat yogurts, pasta, and eat peanut butter! That minimal awareness of how I was ruining my body eventually caught up to me and I paid for it with 12 cavities, a sugar addiction, low mood and energy, and excess weight.

After going through Integrative Nutrition and learning more about the principles of why we crave certain foods, I began to change my eating habits. I saw what worked for my body and what didn't. I noticed that after I ate animal meat I was sluggish and experienced "brain fog." About a month after I became vegetarian I noticed I had more energy, my skin brightened, and my moods stabilized.

A few months later, I came across Dr. Peter D'Adamo's book about the Blood Type Diet. He states that each of the four blood types has a specific roadmap to follow to optimize your health. You can include certain exercises into your life, handle stress in a specific way, and eliminate certain foods from your diet. I am blood type A+ and most type As do better on a vegetarian, plant-based diet.

A study directed by Dr. D'Adamo showed that of the 6,617 individuals who reported their results after following the Blood Type Diet for a period of one month or more, three out of four (71-78%) saw significant improvement in a variety of health conditions. Three quarters of the subjects had an improvement; that is a significant impact! Weight loss was the effect most often observed but a number of reports detailed improvements in digestive function, resistance to stress, overall energy, and mental clarity.

The percentages (71-78%) of patients reporting positive results were consistent across all the blood types. Type O (following a higher protein, lower carb diet) appeared as likely to report positive results as Type A (following a lower fat, plant-based diet) or types B and AB (following a more omnivorous diet).

See **Appendix D** for more on your specific blood type.

Creating a meal plan that works for you will feel empowering, liberating, and will leave you thinking about food in a more positive way. Many people fear food. They are afraid to gain weight and often deprive themselves of "bad" food. I want to invite you to banish that vocabulary. There is no such thing as good or bad, and when you attach that kind of meaning to something, you suffer.

Food is nourishment. Food contains calories and in some cases protein, carbohydrates, and fats. The way you perceive something will create how you feel about it; why not make it fun and see how you feel when you savor food? Why not enjoy food and nourish yourself instead of punishing yourself or attempting to comfort yourself? Change your beliefs and you can create endless possibilities!

Prescription for Mindful Eating and Optimal Energy:

1.   Using your Food Log, journal for one week what you eat and drink. Beverages count, too! Log how you feel just after you eat or drink something, and then how you feel an hour afterward. Pay attention to your energy level: 0 being exhausted/ready for bed, and 10 being ready to jump for joy. Be mindful of your moods. Are you more anxious or agitated? See **Appendix A** for the Handout on Food Log.

2.   What foods/beverages made you feel sluggish? Which ones made you feel energized? Keep track of this and be mindful of how you *felt* since much of our patterns are tied to feeling and can be rewired through positive

memories. People who eat well do so primarily because it makes them *feel* good. You can do the same!

3.   Take a look at the Blood Type Diet and see if you can implement TWO small changes per week. Pay attention to how you feel with those small changes and log it in your journal. This way, you will realize what works and what doesn't work for *your* body.

Chapter 26: I just called to say...I love you

The truth was, I started eating well but I had no idea how to be "loving" to myself. I had listened to so many podcasts and lectures on self-love. What did that even mean? Wasn't someone else supposed to come fill that in?

I would have spurts of treating myself well, but I would revert back to self-sabotaging patterns. At the deepest part of me, I didn't feel worthy of being loved. I was hard on myself. I was still trying to convince my father that I was worthy of his affection, praise, and approval. I rationalized I had a PharmD degree, was studying to be a health coach, and had published an article in one of the major pharmacy magazines, *Drug Topics*.

Wasn't that enough? Wasn't *I* enough?

Dad's mentality was based on hard work. I constantly felt judged, criticized under a microscope. Why was I still fettered by what *he* thought? I was living on my own, paying my bills, flourishing despite lack of support from my family. Yet so much was a mess, and I needed to clean up the debris.

It's easy to say *love yourself,* but let's be honest here. The road to healing is full of ups and downs, anger, frustration, guilt, sadness. Sometimes you look back on your life and say, "Damn, I really did some messed-up, totally crazy shit." I've been there too. In fact, my healing journey of self-love started because of a series of messed-up, dysfunctional relationships.

I started dating a divorcee who was emotionally unavailable, a man who could set a stack of hundreds on fire and still pay for everything. He took me to the Meat Packing District to extravagant candlelit dinners at places like Bagatelle and Catch. He had an apartment in the most expensive area in the city. We would go out and eat delicious, flaky Sea bass with grapefruit and fennel salad, and drink expensive champagne. He told me everything I wanted to hear — that I was beautiful in the candlelight, how much he loved me. We chatted for hours over espresso with anisette. He took me to underground comedy clubs, to the Highline and Chelsea piers. I reveled in being taken care of. Yet I still felt so empty and disconnected from him. Everything was a show — how many bottles of expensive wine we had, how successful he was. I had this gut feeling that he just liked the way I looked on his arm as we pranced around together.

I later dated a narcissistic, manipulative man who lived 5 states away and was also divorced with two children. After that, I was with a controlling, borderline alcoholic who wound up slashing my tires.

Perhaps the worst relationship was the slightly-older divorcee I dated just a few years before writing this book. He was tall, handsome, and all shades of unavailable.

Theme of that time period was: "My name is Christina. I make bad decisions."

It was time to make a good decision. Actually, an enormously brave one. I had "done the personal growth work" over the past couple of months as I was delving into what I stood for, who I wanted in my life, and how I wanted to invest my energy.

I woke up in a guy I was seeing, Matt's bed with a heavy feeling in my heart, one of disappointment and sadness. Immediately I knew what I had to do. Matt and I weren't at the same place—he wasn't ready to share his heart with anyone and I wanted so badly to be with him only. He wanted something different. It took so much strength for me not to cry and to walk away from this person that I had deep feelings for. However much it hurt, I was so proud of myself because in the past I would have just sucked it up, dwelling on what could be in the future, and ignoring every opportunity to meet someone else—someone better.

The night before I left, Matt and I were out at a bar perusing the karaoke list.

"Let's order whiskey!" I said, craving the shot to loosen my nerves and imbue some courage.

"Yeah, sounds good. Let's do that," he agreed, keeping his eyes fixed on the karaoke list as he thumbed through it.

"So what's the deal with us?" I asked him, trying to get a read on him through his eyes as they finally met mine.

"Um...what do you mean?" It was as if I had just asked him to do a calculus problem in the bar. The busty bartender slammed two shots on the table and he smiled at her. "Thanks," he said.

"Um...between us?" I clarified. "We've been seeing each other for a while now. Where do you think this is going?"

"Well, you can date whoever you want, if that's what you mean," he said as he picked up the two shot glasses and faced me.

My stomach turned over and tightened. Fear, anger, and the sudden urge to run away crept into my heart.

"Ha...oh, I'm gonna need another drink," I said as I took back the shot. It burned on the way down, but I loved the pain.

"What's wrong? I told you before, Christina, I'm still somewhat fresh out of my divorce and I don't want anything serious," he explained.

"Mmmhmm. Gotcha. Can I have a Long Island iced tea, please?" I turned from Matt to the bartender.

An awkward pause lingered in the air, then he broke the silence with: "I know what I'm going to sing."

I wanted to cry. I wanted to scream at him and break a glass over his head. *Why don't you love me? What did I ever do to not deserve your love?*

But instead of running out of the bar, I simply let the feeling float past me like a cloud in the sky. I said nothing.

And then it was his turn to sing. *Green Day. Time of Your Life.*

Another turning point, a fork stuck in the road
Time grabs you by the wrist, directs you where to go
So make the best of this test, and don't ask why
It's not a question, but a lesson learned in time

It's something unpredictable, but in the end is right,
I hope you had the time of your life.

So take the photographs, and still frames in your mind
Hang it on a shelf in good health and good time
Tattoos of memories and dead skin on trial
For what it's worth it was worth all the while

It's something unpredictable, but in the end is right,
I hope you had the time of your life.

I laughed as I took a video of him on my phone as he made an ass of himself. The sedation of the whiskey was hitting me hard and I didn't care to ruin the night. I surrendered to the booze and brushed my feelings aside.

Back at his house I fell into his bed, breathless, intoxicated, careless.

Some small voice inside me kept gnawing behind the alcohol. *He can't GIVE YOU WHAT YOU NEED. He told you that at the bar.... Ah, fuck it. Pleasure sounds so good right now. Instant gratification.*

I turned to him and kissed him hard, a mixture of passion and hate. He engulfed my body in an animalistic, provocative, lust-filled way.

"You're so hot, Christina. I want to satisfy you," he said as he spread my legs and hiked my skirt up. He dove into me as I blissfully fell against his body.

And in a silent chatter somewhere in my mind the reel continued.

Empty. Completely. Fucking. Empty. I was betraying myself again....

I woke up next to him in a panic. And in his t-shirt.

"Let's take a shower together," he said, turning to me as my heart sank in my chest.

Haha. Yeah, use my body again. Take my mind, body, soul for all I care. Even though you can't reciprocate. Enough was enough.

"Matt, I can't physically do this," I said finally.

"You mean the sex part? We can just talk if you want," he responded with a wisp of feigned hope.

"No. I can't see you anymore," I said firmly.

"So you don't want to see me anymore?" His eyes looked panicked.

"No...it's not a good idea," I said softly after a long pause.

Finally I had some sense in me. He offered to make me coffee and we talked for a while before I decided to leave. I explained that our conversations were deep and meaningful but his heart wasn't open. Before I left, he pulled me onto his lap and kissed me, saying, "I won't be able to do this for a while." My heart sank knowing he was right. He said something about meeting up for coffee because he enjoyed talking to me, but I didn't count on it.

It shows tremendous growth when you can walk away from someone you truly have feelings for, feel a connection with, yet know they are not in that place to share their heart with you. That day was monumental. I was making choices that would lead me down the right path—the path of truth. It is in the small, everyday choices that our destiny is shaped.

That day I chose self-love. *I trust myself. I love myself.* These were not just words. I embodied the positive affirmations and breathed those principles.

Giving without boundaries means you don't love yourself first. Not speaking your truth suppresses your will and your power. You need to be unconditional with yourself to love another unconditionally.

It was truly a turning point for me.

You can take all of the necessary vitamins, consume wheatgrass shots, drink lemon water, eat clean at every meal, and exercise every day. But something will be missing if you come home to an unfulfilling relationship or constantly feel alone or empty inside. We all need love and connection.

Many factors play into feeling separate or disconnected from one another, including technology and social stigma around vulnerability. Psychologist Barbara Fredrickson has studied love and positive resonance for over two decades and contends that the main mode of sensory connection is eye contact. Since we connect mainly through technology (Facebook, Twitter, iPhone, etc.) eye contact and physical connection are lost.

Physical touch also plays a large role in how we relate to others. Haptics, or the study of touch, is an entire field about how healing the power of physical contact is. Just think of how relaxing and validating it feels when someone touches your shoulder to thank you for something. As a Reiki healer, I channel healing energy to my clients through the power of touch. Physical touch is truly healing for the body, mind, and spirit.

So the question is: If you feel disconnected, how do you reconnect or receive love? Do you get it from yourself? From others?

The first key is to build such a strong foundation of self-love that you do not seek it or rely on it from an external source. Why, you might ask? Isn't my romantic partner supposed to love me unconditionally? That person can provide love to you, yes, but people are only human. We make mistakes at times and are not going to be able to provide consistent acts of love in every moment.

So often what happens in relationships is that we *love* someone up until they do something we don't like. That is not *love*—it is conditional. When you build self-love, you begin having compassion for yourself, which in turn allows you to become more compassionate for others. In this way, you relax and expand your heart to the people around you, connecting to co-workers, family, even strangers. This is the ultimate way to begin to build connection with others.

Second, create opportunities to connect with people face-to-face instead of through technology. It's comforting to understand that we are all craving this connection, but many are afraid to be vulnerable about it. It can be as simple as having lunch with your co-workers instead of sitting at your desk alone. Also, you can choose to make eye contact with your barista at Starbucks instead of texting on your iPhone. This shows care and builds connection, but also allows you to be present in the moment.

These small moments gradually build the muscle of connection that may have been so broken and unconscious. In my experience, I have realized that the more you give your fullest attention to your surroundings and how you interact with those you love, the more enriched those bonds will become. Whatever you focus on will grow.

Ghandi said, "Be the change you wish to see in the world." However, a step before that must be "know thyself" and love thyself before you can truly be an example in the world. So how do you begin to love yourself radically, unconditionally? A step at a time and through turning negative self-talk into loving kindness. The part of you that you ridicule, that you absolutely *hate*, is the part of you that needs the most love and healing. By giving your love to that part, you practice the art of self-care.

Self-care refers to nourishing our physical, mental, emotional, and spiritual well-being through various activities or practices. It is essentially taking allotted time out for yourself to center, ground, and heal any emotional pain or trauma. For example, meditating, watching a funny video on YouTube to ease tension, going for a drive and getting lost in the din of the music, watching the clouds drift by — these are all acts of self-care. Whatever activities resonate with you are the ones you can stick to and repeat as often as you'd like.

There may be a misconception that self-care is equivalent to selfishness, since we are prioritizing our needs and may have to take time away from other plans in our day. However, to love and serve others, we must first tend to ourselves. This is why self-care is so important. It's difficult for us to truly give our attention, love, and care to others when we are depleted. Taking the time to rejuvenate ourselves through these practices allows our energy to become amplified with a current of presence, or aliveness.

We all need self-care, especially during times of high stress. Stress cuts us off from creativity, while self-care renews it. When we are in balance, removed from stress and are happy, we can then fully give our awareness to those we love, creating harmony in this world.

Where in your life today can you create space for a nourishing, fun activity?

Prescription for Self Care:

How are you currently taking care/not taking care of yourself?
-emotionally/mentally
-physically
-spiritually

_____

_____

_____

_____

_____

What action steps can you take to better care for yourself?

_____

_____

_____

_____

_____

_____

Some ideas for you...

Spiritual:
-Cultivate a meditation practice
-Make time for family/friends
-Make time for reflection
-Spend time in nature
-Contribute to causes that you believe in
-Read inspirational literature, listen to inspirational talks

Psychological/emotional:

-Reduce stress as much as possible

-Practice receiving from others

-Write in a journal

-Be curious

-Notice your inner experience: listen to your thoughts, judgments, beliefs, attitudes, and feelings

-Say no to extra responsibilities when you feel overwhelmed

Physical:

-Get a weekly massage

-Reiki energy healing

-Hot yoga, dancing, walking with a friend

-Prepare healthy meals for yourself

-Take the proper supplementation to support mental/physical health

-Take time off and vacations when needed

-Get enough sleep (7-9 hours a night)

-Take time to be sexual/experience pleasure

Emotional:

-Love and cherish yourself!

-Find things that make you laugh

-Allow yourself to cry

-Seek out comforting people, activities, and places

In the Workplace:

-Take regular breaks when needed

-Socialize and connect with peers/colleagues

-Balance your work load so it is not overburdening you

-Speak up when you need help

Be sure to include these activities in your daily routine as much as possible. Love yourself so radically that it pours out of you. Such immense joy will come of this exercise. All it takes is a few small steps.

Chapter 27: I'm bad, I'm bad, I'm really really bad

I had two mentors: Dr. Chawla and Tony Robbins. Tony Robbins would coach me each morning, empowering me to raise the standards in my life as I drove down Atlantic Avenue on my way to work.

At work, Dr. Chawla fed my mind with inspirational videos, books, and websites. She introduced me to the Daily Love, a spiritual website that sent free inspirational emails each day. Every day around 7:15am, the emails popped up in my inbox—things like overcoming fear, living your dream, making suffering optional, constant growth, and stepping into the unknown. Mastin Kipp was the Founder of The Daily Love and had an audio recording of his blog. I'd listen intently, headphones glued to my ears, for any sense of hope. Through the toughest times of my residency, these messages helped kick-start my day. Hearing the audio version of the blog had an even bigger impact on me. All of these powerful voices were my mentors and support system.

I began questioning everything about who I REALLY was. Not the people-pleasing, hardworking Christina, but everything that I had pushed aside a long time ago just to "fit in." I recalled how I told Matt on one of our dates that I was "a dreamer, which was bad." I heard the words come out of my mouth and was shocked. Where had I picked up the belief that I couldn't dream or that it was "bad" to dream? *Society? Family?* I heard my consciousness answer. How many other bullshit beliefs were inside me? I needed to do an entire reassessment of what I stood for, who I was at my core.

I had to figure this out. It wasn't sitting right with me. I made a commitment to unravel who I was at the core, beyond what I had been conditioned to be. Taking on the traits of my father, I had been judgmental, sarcastic, and outgoing. Who was I really?

I began writing in my journal:

Who am I?
I am a person with integrity
Willing to admit when I am wrong
Strong character — will fight for what is right and true
Silly/corny/quirky
Loving/caring/compassionate
Curious, a dreamer, intelligent, intuitive
Willing to look like a fool for love
Good listener, respectful of people's feelings & thoughts
I love hard and I know I will find the one who deserves my love
I want to help others through their food addictions and be a support system for them

First, I needed support. I had never told a soul about my Night Eating disorder but I knew I needed to release it from me to truly heal. It was the most scary, unraveling experience.

I was at my job and had just come back from a Tony Robbins event, "Unleash the Power Within." After going to his event I wanted to change my maladaptive behaviors. I knew I needed support. I couldn't drown in the shame anymore so I called one of my close co-workers into my office. Lenny was a typical Italian male — guarded, stubborn, yet sometimes he gave a glimpse of compassion. I knew I could trust him with my shame.

"Lenny...I have to tell you something and I need help with this. I am not used to being this vulnerable about and I am really ashamed of it. I haven't told anyone about this...." I said, starting to cry.

"What is it? Oh no...don't cry," he said, his eyes softening.

"I get up in the middle of the night and eat. I've been doing this for 7 years now.... I'm really stuck and I need help," I said.

"What do you eat?" he asked.

"Yogurts, chips, whatever I have around." My gaze shifted toward the ceiling as I wiped away thick tears from my eyes.

"Are you kidding me? I've eaten an entire tray of lasagna in the middle of the night! How do you think I got to be this size, Christina?" He raised his voice, breaking into a smile. "Listen, kid, you'll be fine. Just be easy with yourself—you are so damn hard on yourself!"

"Ah...okay, Leonard," I said. I called him Leonard when I was joking around with him. That day a weight was lifted off of me.

Is there someone in your life who you trust? Who do you feel comfortable sharing your secrets with? Is there something you are not speaking up about that is weighing on you? I challenge you to find one person to share this with. Being vulnerable about your struggles will help you lift and release the shame. Everyone has a struggle but not everyone is willing to be vulnerable about it. It may be a silent struggle and when you share your strife, they may open up to you about theirs. This is also how intimacy is established.

First I would ask you—please be gentle with yourself. When you are hard on yourself and criticize, you continue the pattern. When you offer compassion to yourself, you begin to heal. You heal by opening your heart.

Next, do not hold these thoughts or shame in your body. Shame is one of the lowest energy vibrations and does not serve you. You will see in the chapter about energy vibration that anything below courage (200) is false! Do not believe the racket in your mind.

Once you have shared with your safe space, I want you to come back and take notice of how you felt afterward. Did it feel liberating to discuss this? Freeing? Did you bond with this person in a whole new way? Remember that feeling and never give up.

Usually, emotional eating comes from a place of anxiety or disease about something in your current life. Where does the anxiety come from? If you had to look back in time, where in your life did you shut down emotionally and not want to feel? Was it the time you had an argument with your boss or your spouse? Or when you spoke back to your father or mother and got punished?

Take notice of what memories or events come up as you are reading this. Take a few moments to be curious about your unease. Do you know you are not happy in some area of your life and you are FILLING it up with food, alcohol, toxic relationships, drugs, etc.? Did something happen a long time ago that continues to feed the addiction?

A few things that may come up: resistance to doing this activity, fears about what you will discover, the monkey mind wondering why I'm asking you to do this, flipping the pages to the next section. I am asking you to stay with me here. When you can identify, process, and understand these emotions and what triggers them, you can break the cycle.

Like I said, FEAR stands for FUCK EVERYTHING AND RUN. Or the PG version: Forget Everything and Run. Fear is an illusion and everything on the other side of fear is freedom. When you can look at your past as a learning experience and not as a threat, you see that you can create opportunities in the present to shift the way you have been living.

Prescription for Banishing Anxiety:

What right now is creating the most anxiety for you? You can usually pinpoint your fear/anxiety by your "What if" questions. Ex: What if I choose the wrong career path? What if my marriage fails? Are you in a place of discontentment with your job? Are you fearful of what will happen in your relationship? Get curious about what those triggers may be for you and write them down.

_____

_____

_____

_____

_____

As human beings, we crave certainty. We want to know what is going to happen. Will our children be okay? Will I make the right choice to marry someone? And then there are smaller, day-to-day fears, such as: What does he/she think of me? Why am I not being promoted? How will I overcome this addiction?

Tony Robbins said quite accurately, "Quality questions create a quality life." We all have primary questions our subconscious asks and that drive our behaviors. If you ask a disempowering question like "Why am I not losing weight?" your mind will come up with a thousand answers for you. If you say "Why does this always happen to me?" your mind will find that answer as well. Unconsciously, you will perpetuate those thoughts into physical reality. So change the quality of your questions!

My primary question was always, *What is wrong with me?* I grew up thinking I was wrong or bad for expressing my true feelings so I adapted to being a "good girl" to feel safe and accepted. It was not safe for me to speak my truth as I was growing up. I had to keep quiet and do as I was told in order to survive. As I grew older, I found every answer to that question: I developed an eating disorder, denied myself of my true gifts, and chose a career that was not in alignment with my deepest desires, attracted unavailable losers, and did not care about myself. I focused on everyone else's needs to take the focus away from me—and I physically disappeared.

I dug myself so deeply into a career path that I never truly wanted because I thought I had to please my father and make him happy. I gave all of my power away to him. But in the end it made *me* suffer. It was not until I learned how to take my power back through the divine grace of forgiveness that I would be relieved of my pain.

What is your biggest "What if" question? This will lead you to your deepest fears.

_____

_____

_____

_____

_____

_____

_____

Think about what not following your dream/life purpose has *cost* you in health, happiness, and fulfillment. How can you begin to take the steps to move past that fear and step into your power? Write it here.

_____

_____

_____

_____

_____

Chapter 28: Yeah, you shook me all night long!

When you are not connected to your soul, your higher self, you seek to be filled externally. By numbing yourself with these distractions, you avoid being with the deepest part of yourself. It is the ego that wants to keep you small and living a comfortable life. Your soul, or higher self, will be on the other side of you pulling you to fulfill your life purpose, to align with your true self. The ego and the soul can create an inner conflict that leaves you anxious because you innately know you are supposed to be doing something more.

You know what these things are if you are silent enough to be with your thoughts. Sometimes in meditation, harsh memories come up and people want to quit. Sometimes the monkey mind does not let you focus. However, it is in the silence of your own awareness that you will begin to hear what has been harkening you for a long time now.

I did not have a television for 7 years after high school. When I moved out, I was too busy with pharmacy school, social engagements, and going to the gym. After college I moved into an apartment that never had cable installed. Something inside of me was either too lazy to get one or knew I needed to heal myself. Not having a television was the biggest gift for me during that time after college when I was separated from my parents.

Being with my own thoughts allowed me to pray and meditate. I would come home after my residency and light a candle and pray for a resolution with my parents. I would pray that my eating disorder would be healed. I would pray that one day I would be happy, and I asked God for guidance to point me in the direction of my life purpose.

After graduating Integrative Nutrition, I received an email about becoming a Reiki practitioner. Junk mail floods my inbox, as I am sure it does for you! I deleted it. A couple of days later a man whom I met at a Tony Robbins conference suggested I look into energy healing. He said I had a beautiful aura and that I could be a healer. My ego dismissed it. *Who am I to be a healer?* Again, I received an email from The Open Center in New York City about being a Reiki healer.

Okay, enough! I thought to myself. I better look into this—it came to me three times in a week.

What is Reiki, anyway?

The word Reiki is made of two Japanese words—Rei which means "God's Wisdom or the Higher Power" and Ki which is "life force energy." So Reiki is actually "spiritually guided life force energy." If you have breath, you can do Reiki.

Reiki is not taught in the usual sense, but is transferred to the student during Reiki training. This ability is passed on during an "attunement" given by a Reiki master and allows the student to tap into an unlimited supply of "life force energy" to improve one's health and enhance their quality of life. If you can imagine tuning to a radio station, you will only hear the music if that station is tuned in to a certain frequency. When an attunement is given, the frequency of the student is channeled to a high vibration. As long as the healer has a higher vibration than the person being healed, the energy can flow.

Its use is not dependent on one's intellectual capacity or spiritual development and therefore is available to everyone. It has been successfully taught to thousands of people of all ages and backgrounds.

Reiki was discovered by a Japanese monk named Mikao Usui. He would do healings on people by laying his hands over areas of pain. In addition to healing, he would also teach people how to meditate. What he found was that he would do the healing on a person, but they would come back with the same complaint a week or two later. He realized that people had certain karma with each pain and that in order to truly heal, they had to understand *why* they had that pain. To understand your pain and bring love to it will heal that pain. Even if you get a Reiki treatment but avoid understanding the deeper lesson and work to release the pain, you will continue to suffer.

Needless to say — I signed up for the Reiki course and followed the guidance.

This was the point where I became curious about what my pain was telling me. I would soon come to find out.

A perfect example of finding the origin of pain was in one of my patients at the pharmacy I worked at in Queens. Everyone knew of her as the terse, demanding, uptight customer that wanted everything "just-so." She wanted a specific type of generic pill, with what the pill was for written on the prescription label, to be delivered and billed at no charge. When the phone rang and the Caller ID showed her name, everyone cringed.

"You know, I *told* so-and-so NOT to give me the Apotex brand. And I wanted this delivered in the morning! A bunch of idiots! Can't you guys get this right?!"

Everyone yielded to her. When I began working at the pharmacy I knew nothing of her history and spoke with her on the phone one day. I met her with an open mind and gradually got to know her story even though she never physically came into the store. I mentioned to her that I was into healing with essential oils and was a Reiki practitioner, and her energy shifted over the phone.

"Oh...I've tried essential oils. They are absolutely amazing. I love lavender for sleep.... It really helped my anxiety. You know I have had a crazy past, Christine," she said, calling me by the wrong name. She went on to tell me she had been abused as a young child and constantly tried to "escape" through eating emotionally and taking painkillers to numb her feelings. I looked in her chart and knew that the pain was not from anything specific like a physical injury, but from emotional pain.

When traumas happen in life, it's easier to want to block things out than to actually feel them and release them. The problem is, those negative feelings and emotions stay stuck in the body and eventually manifest as a heart attack or diabetes or even an eating disorder. I met this woman with deep compassion, understanding that only people who have been hurt can be hurt others. After that day, she softened and I couldn't help but think that all we really want in life is to be heard and understood.

Another health coaching client of mine had been through Hurricane Sandy and experienced a devastating loss when her husband passed away after he got swallowed up in the basement during the flooding that had occurred. I met her in the vitamin aisle of the Rockaway pharmacy where I worked as she was searching for magnesium.

"What are you using the magnesium for? Do you know what dose you need?" I inquired.

"No. I'm not even sure why I'm taking this…" Her voice trailed off as her gaze followed her confused look. "I think a neurologist gave it to me a while ago," she continued. "I have so many vitamins…. I'm really just trying to lose some weight," she said.

"Well, I am a health coach and a pharmacist. I can help you if you'd like to sit down with me for a consultation sometime soon," I offered. A look of relief came across her face and she agreed to meet with me.

A week later I met with her at a local coffee shop. She had a multitude of health conditions ranging from chronic pain from various car accidents, falling on ice and surgical mishaps, all the way down to allergies, asthma, and acid reflex. The list of herbals and pharmaceuticals she took was lengthy. However, as pharmacists we are trained in Medication Therapy Management, which helps patients with multiple medications and disease states synchronize their medications so they can take them at the appropriate times while reducing side effects. We can also work with their doctors and help minimize the medication load if there are any unnecessary or inappropriate prescriptions on the list.

My plan was to help her with her medications and to understand more of what was preventing her from maintaining a healthy weight. Our bodies are not meant to hold excess weight and what I have found is that the story is always deeper than just intake of excess calories and lack of exercise.

At that time I did not have an office and often went to my clients' homes once I became comfortable enough with them. A few weeks into our sessions, I entered this woman's house. I was overwhelmed with the amount of papers, newspaper clippings, and stacks of old receipts that were piled up all over her kitchen table.

"I'm sorry for the mess. My husband always had so much paperwork piled up everywhere," she nervously explained as I sensed tension in her voice when she mentioned her husband. "And I am still trying to fix up this house. Ever since Hurricane Sandy everything has been a mess here. These contractors said they were coming to look at the shed in the back to fix it and they never did. It is really tough to trust people these days. Would you like a cup of coffee? I have a Keurig." She scrounged through papers looking for the K-cups. She was an endearing woman and always made me feel at home by making me a cup of coffee and offering me pieces of fruit or Greek yogurt.

When I asked her about her eating habits, she was forthcoming that she was an "emotional eater" and could not control her eating, especially at night. She craved sweets and ate ice cream and starchy snacks at night when she got lonely and her mind stopped. Weight

Watchers had helped her in the past since she had to be accountable to someone at the weekly weigh-ins. However, she still found herself back in the cycle of gaining weight over time.

A few things were immediately apparent to me: she needed to clear her space to even begin to work on tending to anything else in her life. She was also holding on to anger towards her husband from Hurricane Sandy, living in the past, and punishing herself by eating emotionally at night when she got lonely. Her mistrust in most doctors, construction workers, and people in general kept her in the vicious cycle of pain and distress. She was constantly fighting her own body or fighting with someone and this pain kept her emotional eating fueled.

My goal in coaching her was to help her get out of her head and connected with her body to eat intuitively. I wanted to help her actually feel her emotions instead of numb them out with food or bury them in a pile of papers in her kitchen.

"I want to help you connect with your feelings…to get out of your head," I explained.

"How do you…feel?" she asked, genuinely.

"Well…you stay connected to what emotion comes up in the moment. You feel it in your heart, then you let it pass like a cloud in the sky. Feelings are temporary but if you do not feel them, they actually fuel your emotional eating," I explained as I recalled countless therapists telling me about this mindfulness technique. "What helps you relax? What do you enjoy doing that gets you out of your head? I want to help you get connected to your heart more. Do you journal?" I asked.

"Yes, I used to paint also. And play the piano," she said, smiling.

"Great! Would you be willing to try one of those activities again?"

"Yes, I could definitely do that. I love the beach, it relaxes me. And I love playing the piano." Her energy shifted to a lighter, more open state.

As our sessions progressed, I worked with her to connect with her emotions, to release the pain. With her permission, I used a release oil in my Reiki energy healing session to alleviate her shoulder and hip pain with positive result. I felt a great deal of energy being pulled in her solar plexus, liver, and pancreas as well as her kidneys. The liver is the area that holds anger and frustration, while the pancreas holds unfinished business. The stomach and solar plexus is the area of the body where pent-up emotions are stored. The kidneys hold stress and tension, since the adrenal glands rest above the kidneys and release cortisol, the stress hormone.

Restoring balance to these areas helps the client feel energized and brings harmony to the emotions that were once dysregulated. It is also a guide for the healer to express to the person being healed where they may need to think about addressing certain areas in their life. In this case, it made sense that these areas in my client were pulling a great deal of energy. The anger, stress, and emotional areas of her life needed to be dealt with on a conscious level through talking through and releasing those painful emotions.

Prescription for Emotional and Physical Pain Relief:

To get more connected to your body, try this mindfulness exercise. For those of you who are more left-brained, this may be challenging, but I am asking you to TRY this exercise to step out of your comfort zone. The idea is to become more present to why you have that pain, whether physical or mental/emotional.

Mindfulness Exercise for Pain Relief:

1. Choose an activity that centers you — whether that is walking meditation, guided meditation, or deep breathing.

2. Light a candle, incense or any other spiritual practice that resonates with you.

3. Pay attention to any tight areas in your body. Do not judge them, just take notice to them. Where are you experiencing pain at this moment? Do you have any tension?

4. Focus on that area and imagine a white light around the area of pain, breathing into that area and sending it positive energy.

5. This may feel odd or uncomfortable, especially if this is an area of continuous pain or frustration for you, but know that you are breaking the pattern and instead of

sending that area fear, you are sending it love and changing the vibrational frequency.

6.   Notice how you feel in this moment. Angry? Sad? Tired? Frustrated? Again, do not judge or label this emotion. Emotions are simply energy in motion and are temporary. Realize they are fleeting and can leave as soon as they come. If you feel tired or nauseous, keep breathing and know that it is the energy releasing.

7.   Keep breathing onto that area and connecting to it, relax into your breath.

As you go on into your day you may feel more centered, less reactive, and even experience less pain in that area of discomfort. Practice this exercise daily and watch your pain dissipate.

Chapter 29: I'm pickin' up good vibrations (Oom bop, bop, good vibrations)

I mentioned previously that your energy vibration creates your reality. Holding onto dense energies like fear, guilt, shame, and resentment lower your 'vibration.' What do I mean by vibration, and why is it so important for health and vitality?

When we typically think of energy and what the universe is made of, we think of atoms and electrons spinning around a nucleus of protons and neutrons. This has been described as the Newtonian Theory of the Universe. However, in the past 100 years, we became aware that we are composed of electromagnetic fields. This explains how we "sense" people's thoughts and energies as we walk into a room. You can feel the energy in a room where there has just been a fight. The energy is tense and you may feel a sense of anger or frustration around that area. Some people are more sensitive to these energies than others, but on a daily basis we are either draining our spirit or replenishing it.

Many of us are constantly depleted by the demands of our job, family, daily commute, etc. You may be in a toxic relationship or unknowingly ingesting harsh chemicals, foods, and beverages. Your vibration, or energy, is strongly correlated to your happiness and physical health. If you have a low vibration, you get sick. Raising your vibration is aligned with health.

How Vibration Affects Health:

-Human cells can start to change (mutate) when their frequency drops below 62MHz.

-58 MHz is the frequency of your body when you have a cold or the flu.

-When candida is present within your body, you vibrate at a frequency of 55MHz.

-52 MHz is the frequency of a body with Epstein-Barr virus present.

-42 MHz is the frequency of a body wherein cancer can appear.

-When the death process begins, the frequency has been measured at 20 MHz.

Wouldn't you agree that this information is worth knowing? Raising your vibration and keeping it high is everything! It is a reflection of your current state of health as well as your contentment and feelings about life. Is there any science behind this stuff? Or is it all just "woo" as many people would say.

High Sense Perception (HSP), or feeling energy with your senses, as Barbara Brennan refers to it, can in fact be measured. Energy cannot be seen physically, but it can be measured. Electrical currents are measured from the brain as EEG (electroencephalogram) waves. Electrical currents from the heart are measured as electrocardiogram (ECG) waves.

As early as 1939, Dr. H. Burr at Yale University found that by measuring the energy of a plant seed, they could tell how healthy the plant would be and how much it would grow. In 1959, Dr. Leonard Ravitz at William and Mary University showed that the Human Energy Field fluctuates with a person's mental and psychological stability. He suggested that there is an energy field associated with these processes, which causes psychosomatic symptoms.

Dr. Bruce Lipton was a pioneer in mind-body medicine, revealing the science of epigenetics, or the study of how the cells in our body are influenced by chemical reactions other than our own DNA sequence. Before Lipton's work, it was thought that we are a by-product of our genetic makeup, or DNA. However, this new school of thought took the control out of the hands of DNA and into the possibility that we are affected by our thoughts and environment.

The mind has visions and thoughts. Your thoughts are based on your programming, and whatever is going on in your life at the moment. Your brain is manifesting an image of that. How is this possible? The brain generates electric signals, and if I put EEG wires on your head, you can see the brain activity printing out.

Your brain is acting as a tuning fork and the broadcast from your brain is not located in your head, so you are like a radio station. Everything in the field vibrates. This idea that we can attract or repel circumstances and people was based upon the research that Lipton conducted.

Lipton started off by placing one stem cell into a culture dish, and then dividing it every ten hours. After two weeks, there were thousands of cells in the dish, and they were all genetically identical, having been derived from the same parent cell.

He manipulated the culture medium—the cell's equivalent of the environment—in each dish. In one dish, the cells became bone, in another, muscle, and in the last dish, fat. This demonstrated that the genes didn't determine the fate of the cells because they all had the exact same genes. The environment determined the fate of the cells, not the genetic pattern. So if cells are in a healthy environment, they are healthy. If they're in an unhealthy environment, they get sick.

Dr. Lipton then took this a step further to link the mind-body connection. "With fifty trillion cells in your body, the human body is the equivalent of a skin-covered petri dish. Moving your body from one environment to another alters the composition of the 'culture medium,' the blood. The chemistry of the body's culture medium determines the nature of the cell's environment within you. The blood's chemistry is largely impacted by the chemicals emitted from your brain. Brain chemistry adjusts the composition of the blood based upon your perceptions of life. This means that your perception of any given thing, at any given moment, can influence the brain chemistry, which, in turn, affects the environment where your cells reside and controls their fate. In other words, your thoughts and perceptions have a direct and overwhelmingly significant effect on cells."

The mind *in love* releases the most wonderful chemicals like dopamine and oxytocin. That same exact mind, when it interprets the world as threatening, releases a whole different set of chemicals. The chemistry released by the brain is a direct connection of the interpretation of the mind.

The chemistry of love, when added to the petri dish, creates cells that grow beautifully. The chemistry of fear cuts down the growth of the system.

The American Psychological Association has recognized that 90% of doctor visits are due to stress, and the stress is due to the interpretation of life not supporting you. If you decide the things that used to bother you aren't bothering you anymore, then you have new chemistry. The mind can decide which thing it's going to focus on. And, whichever thing it focuses on, the chemistry of the brain will be correlated with that thing.

The conscious mind is very slow. "Oh, something over here? Where is it?" And it takes time to find it. The subconscious is so fast, it quickly finds the information and picks out the relevant story.

The subconscious helps you to see those things that are personally connected to you. If you're a person who lives in love, then of course you're going to be moving toward love wherever it is. But if you are a person that lives in fear, then it's going to draw everything into your field—into your attention—everything that could be threatening to you. And all of a sudden, now you have reason to be afraid. Why? You've cleared out everything in your life that would have been good, and you are only looking at the things that are bad.

Neuroscience has shown that 95% of our behavior is directed by our subconscious mind. That means only 5% of what we do on a daily basis is conscious. This is why hypnosis is so powerful—it gets to the subconscious mind, which is running the whole show. There is an analogy of your body being the vehicle and your subconscious mind is the driver. If you don't know how to drive, you will crash the vehicle. In other words, the body will break down if you don't take care of it.

The subconscious mind is extremely powerful and can either guide you to health or keep you in a state of disease. How powerful is your mind? Studies have demonstrated the mind-body connection, especially in the case of psychosomatic illnesses. A researcher named Dr. Ted Kaptchuk studied the response to various placebo treatments in 262 adults with irritable bowel syndrome (IBS). IBS was chosen as the target condition because prior studies have shown it is highly amenable to placebo effects. Also, it is known that IBS is exacerbated or worsened by psychological stress.

The three groups were designed to address three major categories of placebo effects: 1) response to the process of being assessed and observed, 2) response to being given a placebo treatment, and 3) response to the patient-practitioner relationship (placebo acupuncture plus an "augmented" practitioner-patient relationship—with added "warmth, attention, and confidence").

The "placebo effect" is always accounted for in any structured study—from a double-blind randomized controlled trial to a cohort study. The placebo is the fake pill that is given to the subjects of a study to ensure they are unaware of whether or not they are actually getting any treatment or intervention. This allows for a "blinded" opportunity to test the effectiveness of the treatment being tested.

In Dr. Kaptchuk's study, the results were statistically significant, meaning they were relevant enough to be meaningful for the study and for future research. On the symptom severity scale, at three weeks the first group who was assessed and observed without treatment had about a 30-point drop in symptom severity with almost 30% of patients reporting adequate relief; for the placebo treatment group it was 42 points and 44%; and for the augmented group, over 80 points and over 60%, respectively.

What does all this mean? Well, it does confirm what was already known—there are significant placebo effects from the process of being treated, especially with symptoms that are amenable to psychological factors. Even in pharmaceutical studies, a treatment always has to be compared to the placebo to see how effective the drug is. Many times there are clinical improvements in the placebo group, despite the lack of the active ingredient.

How can you begin to change your blood chemistry or your feelings and thoughts? Rewiring the subconscious mind through hypnosis, Buddhist mindfulness techniques or EFT (Emotional Freedom Techniques) are just some of the ways. Realizing that our subconscious thoughts direct our actions is a good first step.

Another brilliant mind, Dr. Masaru Emoto, conducted a study on water in which he performed a series of experiments observing the physical effect of words, prayers, music, and environment on the crystalline structure of water. As he spoke positive, healing words to the water, the water formed a beautiful crystalline structure. As he spoke negative words of hate, the water formed ugly, dissembled patterns.

<<Figure 1>>

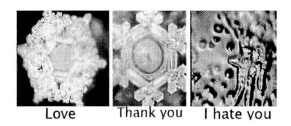

Love   Thank you   I hate you

Our bodies are composed of 70% water and are impressionable to the food, thought patterns, and environment we surround ourselves with. Continual negative thoughts and remarks to ourselves and to each other can have deleterious effects on the body. Speaking kindly to ourselves and to each other has healing effects. Also it is important to drink plenty of filtered water to increase the life force energy throughout your body as well as hydrate your cells and tissues. The recommended daily intake is half your body weight in ounces. For example if you weigh 150 pounds, you should be drinking 75 ounces of water a day, or 9-8 ounce glasses of water.

As I mentioned, everything on this planet originates from energy and emits a certain vibrational frequency. At the molecular level, we are energetic beings with vibrational potential. However, our own physical body emanates an aura, an energy based upon our thoughts, feelings, and emotions. In fact, emotions are a barometer for what is going on within us.

We are all aware of energy fields, even if on an unconscious level. Have you ever walked into a room and felt a denseness to the air as if there were just a fight or an argument that went on there? The harshness or anger may still be palpable in the room. We are able to sense energy even though it is not visible. Nikola Tesla, who studied electricity during the time of Thomas Edison, said, "The day science begins to study non-physical phenomena, it will make more progress in one decade than in all the previous centuries of existence."

Another scientist, Dr. David Hawkins, wrote *Power vs. Nature* and developed the energy vibration scale shown below. Using kinesiology, or muscle testing, he found that when people were in lower energy vibrations of guilt, shame, and fear, they were in a contracted energy state. In other words, they would live in a state of isolation. When a person was in a state of love and spoke a blessing out loud, the muscle testing read 540 on the scale, a level of joy. In this state, people were more expanded, open, and receptive.

Applied Kinesiology (AK) was first described by Dr. George Goodheart after he discovered that taking nutritional supplements would increase the strength of certain muscles. Hostile stimuli would cause those muscles to suddenly weaken. Below our level of consciousness lies infinite body intelligence.

An applied kinesiologist can scan the organs of the body and see where imbalances are. Many chiropractors also use this technique to take a deeper look into imbalances. They can also have the subject hold a supplement, an essential oil, a food, or say out loud a belief to see if they test "strong" or "weak." If a person tests "weak" for any of those things, the kinesiologist can dig deeper into the cause of the imbalance. The body has an EMF, or electromagnetic frequency, that will respond to the EMF of the item or belief in question. This is an objective way to raise your vibration through your own body intelligence!

How does kinesiology work? How do we "test" for a yes or no, true or false statement?

In Hawkins' book *Power vs. Force*, it is described as the following:

1. Have the subject stand erect, right arm relaxed at the side of the body. The left arm is to be held parallel to the floor, elbow straight.
2. Face the subject and place your left hand on his right shoulder to steady him. Then place your right hand on the subject's extended left arm just above the wrist.
3. Tell the subject to resist when you try to push the arm down.
4. Now push down fairly quickly, firmly, and evenly. This tests whether or not the arm can "lock" the shoulder joint against the push.

Assuming there are no other variables such as a problem with the muscle, no presence of dehydration or low blood sugar, and in normal conditions, the muscle will test "strong." If the subject has a negative stimulus such as a chemical sweetener, the arm will drop to his side and test "weak."

As with any scientific experiment, we would like the results to be predictable, repeatable, and universal.

Dr. David Hawkins began his research in kinesiology in 1975. If a subject was given an envelope of artificial sweetener, they tested "weak" while a placebo envelope would produce a "strong" response. His most notable discovery was calibrating a scale of relative truth, by which statements and beliefs could be rated on a scale of 1 to 1000.

Hawkins states, "Each calibrated level represents powerful *attractor fields* within the domain of human consciousness, which serves to explain human behavior."

Application of this scale can be utilized in marketing, advertising, research, and health. Other fields of application are in addictions and self-improvement. This is where I became extremely aware of just how important this scale would be for my own healing and research.

<<Figure 2: Energy Vibration Scale>>

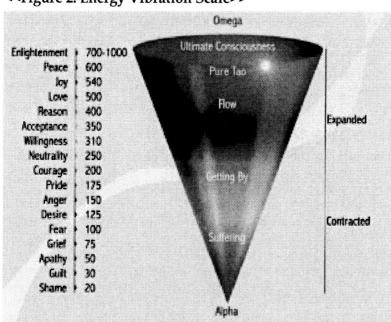

There was evidence that our thoughts produced a physiologic response in the body that caused an energetic shift in our muscles.

Although energy is always fluctuating, this scale proved that different frequencies exist and can be measured.

The average level of consciousness (LOC) of the people in the United States calibrates around 200. However someone at the level of Love (500) or above can raise the energy vibration of 750,000 people below the level of 200. Someone at the level of Willingness can counter-balance 90,000 people below 200. In my wildest dreams I couldn't have imagined impacting that many lives, although I had always had it in my heart to make an impact on the world in a big way. Who knew that just by "being loving" one can make an impact on that many lives? Just by raising your own energy vibration, you can raise and lift others, many of whom you will never meet.

I do not mean *love* in the traditional, conditional sense. Many of us have come to believe love is based upon a feeling of how you relate and exchange with another human being. Hollywood constructs love as being overwhelmed with emotion about another person, but unconditional love is unwavering and does not change dependent upon a person's behavior.

I grew up in a family where love was conditional and based upon what I *did* and how I performed. If I did not do what I was told, I was neglected and given the passive-aggressive treatment. It took a substantial shift in consciousness to heal that trauma. The breakdown started on my bedroom floor. Little did I know it would be the greatest breakthrough toward my healing.

Chapter 30: Let's stay together

One night about 6 months after I left the pharmacy, I broke down. The thoughts came flooding into my mind again. The one pill in the Xanax bottle. The picture being smashed on the deck. I was on my knees on the wood floor of my apartment and I asked God how to take the pain away. I was so fed up with feeling miserable, lonely, and angry.

Forgive them is what came into my consciousness. I breathed into that thought. How could I ever forgive them? *They do not know what they've done. Love them anyway.* My heart filled with compassion for the first time in six months. Yes, they had no idea what they did or why it was wrong on so many levels. But I knew in that moment that I had to begin the process of forgiveness if I ever wanted to free myself.

I came to realize that my parents were extremely afraid of me leaving and they didn't know how else to control me and keep me there. Everyone is a mirror to us and what we do not like in someone else is at the deepest part of us. What we admire in someone else is also within us. If a person directs anger toward you, they may not want to see your light or they may be afraid of it within themselves. If a person is jealous or resentful of you, it may be because they see the gap between where you are and where they are.

Carrying around low vibrational thoughts and emotions does not serve our body and is the source of disease. Yet so many of us carry memories, resentments, and lingering limiting beliefs and "shoulds" about our past. We see the world through a certain lens because of experiences that shaped who we are now, and we carry wounds in our cell tissue from events that took place in our past. Many of these unconscious beliefs are so deeply seated in us that we may not even be aware of them. Ex: Unhealed childhood experiences or traumas which lead to thoughts of "I am not enough"=guilt, or "I am bad"= shame. If not released and healed, these toxic thoughts linger on well into adulthood.

Dr. Hawkins points out that the two greatest spiritual growth barriers seem to be at level 200 (courage) and 500 (love). Two hundred, the level of courage, represents a profound shift from destructive and harmful behavior to life-promoting lifestyles; everything below 200 makes one go weak using kinesiology. Currently, approximately 78% of the world's population is below this significant level. The destructive capacity of this majority drags down all of mankind without the counterbalancing effect of the 22% above 200. Because the scale of consciousness is logarithmic, each incremental point represents a giant leap in power.

A person's LOC remains rather steady throughout their lifetime. Emotions come and go like the passing wind, but a person's LOC is governed by specific energy fields in the nonlinear, spiritual domain, which generally doesn't waver. Over the course of a lifetime, the average person's LOC will change approximately 100 points; this is not a statistical derivation, but an average discovered through Dr. Hawkins' kinesiologic research. However, it is possible for an individual (such as a spiritual aspirant) to have their LOC jump (or drop) hundreds of points in a single lifetime.

Your personal energy field can be light or heavy depending on:

- Your personal daily choices and habits
- The health of the environment you're in at work and at home
- The thoughts and feelings you have about yourself and others
- How judgmental you are of others
- If you have a strong 'inner critic'
- If you use guilt and shame to control other people
- The foods/beverages you ingest

What are the different levels and how do you know where you reside primarily? See if you can identify with what your feelings are in a typical week by looking in the LOC below:

The Levels of Consciousness (LOC):

Shame (20)
According to Hawkins, this is one step above death. At this level, the primary emotion one feels is humiliation. It's not surprising that this level, being so close to death, is where most thoughts of suicide are found. Those who suffer from sexual abuse often calibrate here, and without therapy they tend to remain here.

Brene Brown, a professor and researcher who studied shame, vulnerability, and courage, had an incredible, moving TED talk on these topics. She spoke about her extensive research on shame and how it tied into the fear of being vulnerable. We have this fear that if someone 'finds out' what we did, we won't be accepted or lovable. In reality, when people are vulnerable it forms connection. It takes courage to be vulnerable, but speaking out loud about what has been holding you back and weighing on you raises your vibration.

Along my healing journey, I attended a Landmark course and was amazed at the strength of the people who got up to the microphone and shared their story. The course was called the Forum, similar to ancient Greek amphitheaters where people would speak openly about a topic. However, many people went up to the microphone to reveal their story and have their pain resolved by talking it through with the coach, Jerry. He made fun of himself by saying he was *all teeth no eyes.* He had squinty eyes and big, protruding teeth.

One woman approached the microphone looking extremely nervous. "So…I have this thing that I want to resolve…" she said as her voice cracked and tears began to fall from her beautiful almond-shaped eyes.

"When I was four…." She couldn't finish the sentence, but tried again.

"When I was four…I was raped by my brother's friend…"

My heart felt like it lodged in my throat.

"I see. And what meaning did you make out of that event?" Jerry asked slowly and patiently.

"I don't know. That it was my fault?" she asked through broken tears.

"Yes, that you were a little girl and it was your fault for getting raped," he said. "But you aren't four anymore, are you?" She shook her head. "Yet you still blame yourself, right?"

She nodded. "I wanted my parents to be there to protect me and they weren't! I didn't deserve it...." Her anger quickly turned to sadness.

"No you didn't, but do you want to complete this thing now? We can clear this away for you. What would you say to that little girl if you could be with her now?" he asked.

"I would say not to worry and it isn't your fault." She sobbed.

"I want to hear you say it loud and clear for everyone to hear."

"I WOULD SAY IT ISN'T YOUR FAULT!!!" she said loudly and then broke into a smile.

"Good. You don't have to make meaning out of that event anymore. You can know that you did not deserve that and it is not your fault," Jerry said.

I commended how brave this woman was for being vulnerable enough to share her shame with the group. What I realized was that once shame is released, it no longer has a grip on you. It no longer binds you because we all experience shame. We are all afraid that our secrets will be found out and that we will be rejected or unlovable, so we keep it to ourselves.

The reality is, the more vulnerable you are, the faster you heal and the more connection you form with others. You also allow others to express their vulnerability and thus help them heal. That was my intention with this book — to tell my healing story so other people may also start or continue on their journey to healing.

Looking in the mirror and into the past can be scary. I promise you that if you complete the process, you will release heaviness that has been weighing on you. Your creator wants you to be happy, alive, and thriving.

The way out of the pain is to dive straight into it, even if you're scared. In my therapy group, we had spoken about several Buddhist concepts of observing our thoughts with compassion and non-judgment. I was so emotionally scarred and hard on myself. I nit-picked at everything I did wrong. The Loving Kindness Meditation in the Appendix of this book was one of the healing modalities I used during that time. The idea is to give yourself unconditional love, then offer it to a pet/loved one, then to extend that love to even your enemies or those who trigger you. The more you can cultivate compassion and love for yourself, the more your heart will soften for others, even enemies.

See the Release Process in **Appendix B** to help release shame.

Guilt (30)

Not too far from shame is the level of guilt. When one is stuck in this level, feelings of worthlessness and an inability to forgive oneself are common. This translates as "I did something bad" and is toxic to a person's growth and ability to reach for the things they want. Many times others will "make" the person feel guilty and their perception is that external forces are controlling their life. It takes ownership and strength to move up the vibration scale. If you constantly felt guilty, how do you think you would act? Would you try to reach for your dreams? Would you be in a loving relationship? You would not think you deserve to be happy at this level. Breaking through that false core belief is imperative for graduating up the scale.

Apathy (50)

The level of hopelessness and despair; this is the common consciousness found among those who are homeless or living in poverty. At this level, one has abdicated themselves to their current situation and feels numb to life around them.

Grief (75)

Many of us have felt this at times of tragedy in our lives. However, having this as your primary level of consciousness, you live a life of constant regret and remorse. This is the level where you feel all your opportunities have passed you by. You ultimately feel you are a failure.

Fear (100)

People living under dictatorship rule, or those involved in an abusive relationship find themselves at this level. There is a sense of paranoia here, where you think everyone is out to get you. Suspicion and defensiveness are common.

Desire (125)

Desire is a major motivator for much of our society. Although desire can be an impetus for change, the downside is that it leads to enslavement to ones' appetites. This is the level of addiction to such things as sex, money, prestige, or power. A strong level of needing to be important or validated may hinge on desire.

Anger (150)

As one moves out of Apathy to Grief and then out of Fear, they begin to want. Desire that is not fulfilled leads to frustration which leads to Anger. This anger can cause us to move out of this level or keep us here. Most of the time anger is directed toward the self for not being where they would like to be. There is much resistance to the present moment here.

Pride (175)

According to Hawkins, since the majority of people are below this point, this is the level that most people aspire to. It makes up a good deal of Hollywood. In comparison to Shame and Guilt, one begins to feel positive here. However, it's a false positive. It's dependent upon external conditions such as wealth, position, or power.

Courage (200)

This is the level of real empowerment. It is the first level where you are not taking life energy from those around you. Courage is where you see that you own your power and are not affected by your external conditions. This empowerment leads you to the realization that you are a steward unto yourself, and that you alone are in charge of your own growth and success. This is what makes you inherently human: the realization that there is a gap between stimulus and response and that you have the potential to choose how to respond. Cultivating a meditation practice is the way to widen the gap.

Neutrality (250)

Neutrality is the level of flexibility. To be neutral, you are, for the most part, unattached to outcomes. At this level, you are satisfied with your current life situation and tend not to have a lot of motivation towards self-improvement or excellence in your career. You realize the possibilities but don't make the sacrifices required to reach a higher level.

Willingness (310)

These are those people around you who are perpetual optimists. Seeing life as one big possibility is the cornerstone of those operating here. No longer are you satisfied with complacency—you strive to do your best at whatever task you've undertaken. You begin to develop self-discipline and willpower and learn the importance of sticking to a task until you complete it.

Acceptance (350)

If Courage is the realization that you are the source of your life's experiences, then it is here where you become the creator of them. Combined with the skills learned in the Willingness phase, you begin to awaken your potential through action. Here's where you begin to set and achieve goals and to actively push yourself beyond your previous limitations. Up to this point you've been generally reactive to what life throws at you. Here's where you turn that around, take control, and become proactive.

Reason (400)

The level of science, medicine, and a desire for knowledge. Your thirst for knowledge becomes insatiable. You don't waste time in activities that do not provide educational value. You begin to categorize all of life and its experiences into proofs, postulates, and theories. The failure of this level is you cannot seem to separate the subjective from the objective, and because of that, you tend to miss the point. You fail to see the forest because you're tunnel-visioned on the trees. Paradoxically, Reason can become a stumbling block for further progressions of consciousness.

Love (500)

Only if in the level of Reason you start to see yourself as a potential for the greater good of mankind, will you have enough power to enter here. Here is where you start applying what was learned in your reasoning and you let the heart take over rather than the mind. You live by intuition. This is the level of charity — a selfless love that has no desire except for the wellbeing of those around them. This is where the welfare emotions are — compassion, forgiveness, and acceptance. Gandhi and Mother Theresa are examples of people who were living at this level. Only 0.4 percent of the world will ever reach it.

Joy (540)

This is the level of saints and advanced spiritual people. As love becomes more unconditional, there follows a constant accompaniment of true happiness. No personal tragedy or world event could ever shake someone living at this level of consciousness. They seem to inspire and lift all those who come in contact with them. Your life is now in complete harmony with the will of Divinity, and the fruits of that harmony are expressed in your joy.

Peace (600)

Peace is achieved after a life of complete surrender to the Creator. It is where you have transcended all and have entered that place that Hawkins calls "illumination." Here, a stillness and silence of mind is achieved, allowing for constant revelation. Only 1 in 10 million (that's .00001 percent) of people will arrive at this level.

Enlightenment (1000)

This is the highest level of human consciousness where one has become like God. Many see this as Christ, Buddha, or Krishna. These are those who have influenced all of mankind.

Hawkins' *Power vs. Force* and his associated map of consciousness has been a groundbreaking work for those interested in human consciousness development. In this continuum, we can clearly see where we as individuals function and where we can arrive. A view into what could be our potential is inspiring.

It's interesting to note that according to Hawkins, everything around us can affect our level of consciousness: the music we listen to, the people with whom we associate, the books we read, the shows we watch, etc. We are all at different levels of consciousness and are functioning according to the light and knowledge we've obtained. This has helped me to better understand what drives people and why they make specific choices.

How can we raise our LOC or "vibration?" What level are you at currently? Take an honest inventory. The key to raising your vibration is a willingness to do so. Hawkins stated that most people have an LOC set point and do not fluctuate beyond a mere 5 points of that. However, passing through to the higher levels can be achieved through cultivating compassion, forgiving, and coming to an acceptance of all that is around you.

Remember I mentioned that raising your energy vibration aligns you with health and true happiness, which is fulfillment? The idea is to be in the higher vibrations to be in alignment to heal and be fully fulfilled.

Prescription to Raise Your Energy Vibration:

First realize that what you FOCUS on, you FEEL. In Sanskrit, your *drishdi*, or focus, is dependent on where you will end up. In yoga, if you focus on the floor, you will wind up there. Hone your *drishdi* to think positive thoughts. I am not telling you to ignore negative thoughts. That is unrealistic. But allowing the thoughts to come and to laugh at how ridiculous they are is possible. You can say to yourself, *Oh there I go again. My ego is telling me false beliefs.* Then insert a positive one.

One of the most powerful things I did for myself was sit quietly by my mirror, staring at my reflection. I told myself *I love you. You are so beautiful. Never forget how beautiful you are…* I would stay there for at least 5 minutes just looking into my eyes with compassion. Gradually this melted away much of my self-doubt and low self-esteem, and I soon felt strong and comfortable in my own skin.

Once you have the self-love and acceptance part going, how do we deal with the rest of the world? It may be more simple dealing with your own self-love, but people can be *cruel!* Often we react to people because they trigger something in us. Why does our brain automatically go to reaction mode? Your habitual response to people usually follows the schematic below:

THOUGHTS lead to **EMOTIONS** which trigger **REACTIONS**

We get triggered emotionally because of our underlying beliefs and perception about what that person said. If you believe you are fat and someone makes a comment like, "That dress looks tight on you, but you look great!" Your amygdala, or emotional brain, will be wired to protect you. You may respond in an angry fashion and lash out because your core belief is that you are fat. If someone else who did not have that underlying belief was in the same situation, they may laugh it off because they know it isn't true. The same goes for other comments about how smart, pretty, or successful we are. Everyone has their trigger points that show up in order to be healed.

How can we slow down and allow comments to roll off our back? You can utilize meditation to slow these thoughts down and widen the gap between those thoughts. Think about being seated on a riverbank and watching boats go by. The boats represent thoughts. You can choose to focus on the boats and jump on them to be carried upstream. Every time a boat passes you are tempted to get back into old thought patterns and react the same old way. You can choose to get on the boat and get stuck in the upstream current, or you can slow down the boats and just see them passing by. Of course you still have thoughts, but you do not react to every single one. It does not trigger you to react in old ways.

Remember, we cannot control other people, but we can control how we *respond* to other people. Instead of seeing our spouse/boss/children as a source of our unhappiness, we take personal responsibility for our own energy and feelings. The two options we always have are choice and awareness.

Many of us want to take credit for all of the good things in our life. We own it and are proud of those things! But we put responsibility on other people when our life has gone down a destructive path. It is our parents' fault that we always choose a dysfunctional relationship. It is our bosses' fault that we are stuck in a job where we are not really appreciated or heard. It takes a lot of courage to look in the mirror and take ownership for all aspects of your life. You have created this!

Another way to raise your vibration is through ingesting high vibrational foods. Food is a key pleasure in our life! It is okay to use food to nourish your body and indulge every so often. Remember your body is in physical form and is made of 70% water. Nourishing it with high vibrational foods and positive thoughts will allow you to heal.

The Ancient Greeks believed that eating high-energy foods helps us reach higher consciousness and better connect with our higher source. This is one of the reasons many ancient philosophers and healers such as Plato and Pythagoras were vegetarians.

What are high vibrational ("high energy") foods? They are plants and fruits from the earth that vibrate or are in alignment with our true nature. For example: organic fruits and vegetables, legumes, and nuts. Essentially, they come from the earth. Eating these types of foods results in health and harmony in the body, whereas foods with a low vibrational quality result in sickness and disharmony.

We can derive so many healing benefits from the foods we choose to consume each and every day. It is truly medicine, and we can choose to eat high-quality, nutrient-dense foods to prevent illness.

See **Appendix F** for List of High and Low Vibrational Foods

Microwaving food changes the life energy of that food. Instead, you can bake or broil the food to heat it.

I have found that negative thought patterns and consuming too much sugar, caffeine, and "low quality/low vibrational" foods leads to weight gain, low energy, and anxiety. We deserve to wake up feeling vibrant and alive. This starts in the physical form by nourishing your body.

As you begin to raise your vibration, you will notice a few things:

- You will begin to attract positive people in your life as the frequency of negative people will not match yours anymore.
- You may have a strong desire to help the world in some deep and meaningful way.

- You will feel a lightness in your body and even a spontaneous sense of joy.
- You will realize that when people are reacting to you, they are really projecting their fears.
- You notice an enormous amount of compassion that manifests as an expansion in your heart for all creatures and the world in general.
- You nourish your body with healthy foods because it makes you feel energized, positive, and refreshed.
- Material things do not draw your attention anymore; instead you focus on cultivating your dreams and ideas.

Chapter 31: Oh without you now, this is what it feels like

I looked and saw that for much of my life I stayed in low vibrational thought patterns that were perpetuating my eating disorder. When I came across the chakra (energy) system, I found there were other patterns I needed to break.

I was so afraid to speak my truth, especially in the face of a male authority figure. I never wanted to rock the boat for fear of having someone withdraw from me. Relationships with guys were hot and cold—I would get very close to them and then push them away because I couldn't trust myself. I wanted the certainty of love in my life but I couldn't trust myself to choose the right people to give it.

Perpetuating the same pattern means there is a core belief that creates an emotion in your body and will attract the same type of circumstance over and over until you learn the lesson. Ignoring an illness and masking symptoms with prescription drugs will never heal you. The same goes for unhealthy relationship patterns. Something is motioning for you to pay attention to heal the trauma. There may be energy blocks and limiting beliefs within you that prevent you from healing core wounds from childhood.

I came across the chakra system again during my residency. Caroline Myss spoke about how our energies get taken in and are governed by the chakra system, which consists of 7 energy fields. Everyone has an energy field or aura that surrounds us and interpenetrates the physical body. This energy field is intimately associated with health. I mentioned High Sense Perception in a previous chapter. HSP is a way of perceiving things beyond the normal range of human senses. With it, one can see, hear, smell, taste, and touch things that cannot normally be perceived. High Sense Perception is a type of "seeing" in which you can perceive a picture in your mind without the use of your normal vision. It is sometimes referred to as clairvoyance.

With HSP, the mechanism of psychosomatic illness lies within the energy field. Many times the source of illness comes from psychological or physical trauma, or a combination of the two. Congested chakras reveal where the source of illness is.

Every chakra acts to vitalize each auric body and thus the physical body. The chakras are each associated with a major endocrine gland and nerve plexus. For example, the first chakra is associated with the adrenals, which deal with stress hormones such as cortisol and adrenaline. If this area is congested, a person may experience a multitude of symptoms such as ADHD, acne, or an autoimmune disease such as psoriasis, rheumatoid arthritis, etc.

When a chakra is energized and balanced, it will exhibit a clear vibrant color in the energy field and will rotate evenly in a clockwise direction. A congested chakra will have a dull hue in the energy field and may be stagnant or rotating counter-clockwise if undercharged.

Functions of the Chakra System:

Chakra	Endocrine Function	Area of Body Governed	When balanced	When blocked, either excessive or deficient
1	Adrenals	Kidneys, spine	Strong will to live, grounded, feeling safe	Acne, arthritis, autoimmune diseases, constipation Excessive: overly possessive; fearful parent Deficient: homeless; ungrounded; victim
2	Gonads	Reproductive system	Ability to express emotions, Sense of abundance and well-being, Healthy sexual function	Fertility problems, urinary problems, hip/pelvic/low back pain Excessive: manipulative, controlling, lustful, addictive Deficient: co-dependent, martyr, submissive, doesn't feel anything, shut down
3	Pancreas	Gallbladder, stomach, liver	Self worth, confidence, esteem, clear thinking	Digestive problems, diabetes, eating disorders, controlling/critical behavior Excessive: egotistical, self-absorbed; ambitious self-driven warrior, desire to take control Deficient: poor self-

				worth; sensitive servant; feels disliked; martyr; needing to "do" all the time
4	Thymus	Heart, blood, circulatory system	Love, ability to forgive, joy and inner peace	Congestive Heart failure, anger, bitterness Excessive: inappropriate emotional expression; poor emotional boundaries Deficient: ruthless, no heart, can't feel emotions
5	Thyroid	Bronchial and vocal apparatus, lungs	Self-expression, speaking the truth	Under/overactive Thyroid, TMJ, ADHD, neck/shoulder pain, ulcers Excessive: willful, controlling, judgmental, hurtful speech Deficient: lacking faith, unable to creatively express, silent child
6	Pituitary	Ears, nose, nervous system, lower brain	Clear thinking and decision-making, intuition	Migraines/headaches, blurred vision, hearing loss Excessive: overly intellectual; overly analytical Deficient: unclear thought; deluded
7	Pineal	Upper brain	Pure bliss, self knowledge	Confusion, fear of alienation Excessive: cult leader,

			and divine connection	ego maniac Deficient: no spiritual inspiration/aspiration

If your answer is YES to any of the following questions, you may be blocked or have a congested chakra in the corresponding energy center:

1. Root Chakra –Do you feel stuck in your current life situation? Did you recently experience a traumatic event, family problems, death of a loved one, or other major life change?

2. Sacral Chakra – Do you feel unmotivated for life especially towards exercise or sex? Do you have an addiction or eating disorder?

3. Solar Plexus Chakra – Do you have a sugar addiction, eating disorder or insomnia? How well do you set boundaries with others?

4. Heart Chakra – Do you feel disconnected to yourself and others with an inability to love? Are you compassionate toward yourself and others?

5. Throat Chakra – Do you have attention deficit disorder? Feel isolated, nervous/anxious? How well do you speak your truth?

6. Third Eye Chakra – Do you have trouble making decisions and feel confused and unable to follow your intuition?

7. Crown Chakra – Do you feel disconnected spiritually and that you cannot find your direction or purpose?

For example, a 3rd chakra imbalance comes from lack of healthy boundaries, meaning you typically say "yes" when you mean "no," betraying your true feelings. I used to do this because I felt so guilty saying no to people. I had weak boundaries and I would do almost anything people asked me to.

Many people are caregivers/healers and are selfless people! It is a beautiful thing to be selfless and serve others. However, there needs to be an energy exchange, a giving and receiving. Often people-pleasers will have the mentality that they need to help others before helping themselves. Think about it, how can you serve and give to others if you are depleted? I liken it to the airplane oxygen mask—you are supposed to put on *your own mask* before putting it over the child or other person you are with.

Other people lose energy from constant anger and frustration because they are resistant to what is in the present moment. These are the people you see screaming at customer service or exploding at their spouse for something insignificant. When you resist life, you create pain, which blocks life-force energy and ultimately leads to disease. This is a 1st chakra block along with a 7th. You are unwilling to accept the present moment, to feel connected to the earth and a higher power.

Accepting the present moment and realizing that the only thing we can control is how we respond is the way to let go of anger. You can feel the anger and release it, but if you do not *process it* you, will *project it.* Also, blaming and lack of forgiveness blocks energy and leaves you powerless. This is a 4th chakra block in the heart center. Taking ownership and responsibility of your part in the situation does not excuse bad behavior of others, but allows you to take your power back.

When you blame others for your pain, you are acting out the role of a victim. Seeing illness as a gift and opportunity to correct the imbalances in your life will allow you to heal.

Many caregivers and mothers wind up having a 3rd chakra imbalance. Men can have a solar plexus tear also! I have worked with many people who give too much of themselves, so much that they forget about taking care of themselves. They are unable to set healthy limits on how much of themselves they give to a project for their boss or the needs of their child, and they wind up suppressing or ignoring their own needs. Or, as in many eating-disorder cases, people seek approval from others to be validated for their own self-worth.

One of my clients from the pharmacy wanted to lose weight after she was diagnosed with diabetes. I met her in one of the diabetes classes I taught and formed a strong bond with her.

She was a beautiful African American woman who wore big costume jewelry and had long nails. She had recently developed Type 2 Diabetes and her A1C, the measurement of blood sugar over a 3-month period, was 9% upon diagnosis. The American Diabetes Association Guidelines set a target of an A1C less than 7% to prevent long-term disease complications such as nerve damage, kidney damage, amputation, and blindness. Typically, this woman would be immediately put on insulin; however her doctor had given her the chance to lower her A1C with oral medication and lifestyle modification, meaning diet and exercise.

Upon speaking with her, I got her history—the medicine she took, her blood sugar levels, what she loved to do. She seemed like a content, pleasant woman with not much stress in her life. After retiring from the Port Authority she was resting on a comfortable pension and enjoying life with her husband. However, she also spoke about a friend who took a great deal of her energy.

"Yes, I will spend an hour on the phone with Barbara. I don't even have to talk! She just loves to talk and complain..." she said, smiling politely.

I picked up on the energy that she tended to give her power away easily to people because she wanted to be liked, thus why she had so many friends. Also, this woman Barbara was sucking the energy out of her by keeping her on the phone for an hour at a time.

"Do you get off the phone at times and feel depleted?" I asked her. "Lacking energy?"

"Oh yes. I will get off the phone and take a nap right away," she answered.

"I thought so. This woman might be draining your energy. What if you cut your conversations down to 10 or 15 minutes instead of an hour? That way you can still keep your friendship but also take care of your needs?" I offered.

"Wow...you are right. I never connected the two. I'm always tired after I get off the phone with her. I'm going to try that next time," she said.

For the rest of our sessions, she would bring up this woman Barbara and thank me for helping her minimize her exposure to the toxic friend.

If you don't set healthy limits with people, they will drain your vital energy. There is a way to do this so that you do not feel guilty or feel like you are hurting the other person. Take ownership of *your* feelings and do not project. For example, if you are feeling tired and want to leave the table at dinner, you could say something like, "Listen, I'm feeling tired and need to excuse myself. I'll catch up with you later." It sounds simple but for someone who is not used to setting boundaries and honoring their feelings and body, this is tremendous for energy conservation. This is a way to take care of yourself.

Another woman who had diabetes came to me after her husband picked up my business card at a local juice bar in Queens. She was a beautiful woman who had developed diabetes after her third child. Her main concern was her anxiety. She had tremendous anxiety that manifested as sharp, radiating pain down her neck, and she had suffered panic attacks in the past.

Growing up, she had to parent herself because her mother was constantly out partying during her teen years. Looking for stability, she started dating an older guy and made him the center of her universe. She loved the fact that he was dependable and had a stable family, something she lacked in her own life. She began staying home and stuffing her face with pasta, cookies, cake, and other yummy Italian food.

She went from 100 pounds to 160 pounds, which was not healthy for her 5'3" frame. Unconsciously, she was hiding herself so no other man would look at her. She held on to a tremendous amount of guilt and shame because of her family's past, and she had it in her mind that she needed to make herself invisible to other men so she could keep her new boyfriend. All of this served her because she hid herself and kept her boyfriend, even though she had gained the weight.

After getting married to this boyfriend and having three children, she became sick. She suffered a massive panic attack and was finally pushed against a wall. Her husband then found my card.

Upon talking with her, she told me she was a "guilty" person and did not want to rock the boat by speaking her truth to her husband. She had always feared speaking up to him about anything because she didn't want him to leave her. She embodied the ideal of a "perfect wife" and tended to the children, did what she was told, and kept the house in order.

She and I were cut from the same cloth—we had given our power away to other people (solar plexus imbalance) and wound up sick. Instead of an eating disorder, she developed an actual physical disease—diabetes. Her body was rejecting itself, since this type of diabetes weakened her immune system.

My goal was to help her heal by realigning with what she truly craved along with meeting her health goals of lowering her blood sugar to a healthy level and nourishing her body with the proper food and supplementation. She started an exercise routine and gradually learned to set healthy boundaries with her family, something she had never done before. She stopped blaming everyone else for her discontentment and took her power back.

Prescription to Align Your Energy Centers (Chakras):

1. Encourage positive thought patterns
2. Get out in the sun for at least 10 minutes a day
3. Eat foods that contain each of the seven color energies
4. Do meditation and/or yoga
5. Wear gemstones or place them in your environment
6. Practice aromatherapy
7. Listen to music and dance
8. Listen to high vibrational toning & sounds like Tibetan Bowls or gongs
9. Decorate your home or office with positive colors; surround yourself with color (calming colors in bedroom, stimulating colors in workplace)
10. Receive Reiki energy healing

Chapter 32: Don't turn around, you don't wanna see my heart breakin'

The third chakra controls your will, self-esteem, and self-worth. When the third chakra is blocked, you feel insecure, powerless, and out of control. Once you begin to own your power, you will find it easier to reach for the things you want that bring you long-term fulfillment. The solar plexus chakra connects with the fifth chakra, which is how you direct your will to speak your truth. When the solar plexus chakra (3rd) is strong and the energy can move through the heart chakra (4th) up to the throat chakra (5th), a person easily speaks their truth.

The heart is the center of the chakra system and the gateway from the lower three chakras (root, sacral, solar plexus) to the top three chakras (throat, third eye, and crown). The lower three are everything in the physical realm and the top three connect to your spiritual self. Every situation can be healed through the heart.

Most of us live in our ego, in the mind where there are thousands of thoughts darting in and out. Should I take the job? Do I really need help or should I ignore the problem? Can I make this relationship work? Is it worth it?

I can recall so many times that I went against my gut feeling only to find out it was spot on. Some may call this intuition, others may call it a gut feeling or just a *knowing* that transcends the mind. If you listen to your heart, it will always direct you to the right path.

God speaks to you through your heart. You *know* the answers; you just have to quiet the mind to listen.

Most of us don't want to hear the answers the heart tells us. This is your soul urging you to take care of yourself, to escape a toxic relationship or job. When you listen to your heart, you may not like the answer. There is a lot of uncertainty that goes along with following your heart and most of us crave certainty and safety. It's scary to hear the answers. However, your heart is a compass to your true happiness.

When I was in my last year of pharmacy school trying to figure out what I wanted to create for my life, there was something pulling at me. I tried to ignore the inner voice, stuffing it down with food. I didn't want to hear the truth: that I was not meant to work at my father's pharmacy. How unsafe and uncertain would that be for me? I had worked at the same place for 10 years and had never gone on a job interview. I was a hard worker but I never had to face the real world of a Human Resources department and an organizational structure.

There was a yearning deep within me to make an impact on the world and although I was scared to death, I needed to follow that voice. Tying that emotion to a greater purpose helped me get through the fears, the doubts, and the verbal abuse. It takes courage to be yourself, to follow your heart's desire and take a leap of faith.

What I have found with myself and with so many others is that when you speak your truth with love, anything is possible. Broken relationships get restored, healings happen, and a deeper gratitude for life is revealed. So many people are afraid to speak the truth because it's easier to pretend everything is okay. I pretended for a long time that I was happy and satisfied with life. On the inside I was dying and miserable. It was only when I was able to speak my truth that I felt free and a deep sense of relief.

I used to go to aerobics classes at a gym in Howard Beach when I first started my residency. All of the women in the class were typical Italian women. Many were housewives that left their children with the babysitter outside of the room. We used to go into the sauna to relax our muscles after the gym class.

One day I was talking to a woman, Rose. The holidays were approaching and I asked her what her plans were.

"I'm going to have a quiet Thanksgiving at home with my husband. We used to get together with all of the kids, but I'm not talking to my daughter right now," she said.

"You have two daughters, right? If you don't mind me asking, what happened that you aren't seeing them for the holiday?"

"My older daughter and I really don't get along. We always butt heads. Every time I try to talk to her, she feels attacked. I'm not trying to control her, but I want to help her with her problems. She thinks I get too involved in her life. We had a fight a few months ago because she curses me out every time I try to talk to her. It was the last straw — she is so ungrateful and rude."

"I can understand where both of you are coming from," I said. "How do you feel about spending the holidays without her?"

"It really hurts me…" she said, starting to cry.

"Have you told her that?" I asked.

"I can't go back. She has no respect for me. She needs to learn her lesson." Her voice tightened.

"What if she was just as hurt as you and wanted to connect with you again? What if it was all just a miscommunication between you two? I know because my dad and I have the same dynamic. He pushes my buttons so much, but I came to him with an open heart and forgave him. Now things are shifting."

"Ah…I'm too hurt," she said, wiping her tears away.

"Okay. When you are ready, you will open your heart to her again." I left the sauna and prayed for her to reconcile with her daughter.

A week later I returned to the class. Rose had such a look of relief on her face, one much less tense than last week in the sauna. I had an inkling that she had reconciled. After class, we went into the sauna again.

"Christina…thank you so much for last week. I opened my heart to my daughter and apologized for impeding too much in her life. I told her I loved her and just wanted the best for her. She met me with open arms and now we are having Thanksgiving together," she said, filled with joy.

"Oh I am so happy for you, Rose!" That was the first time I truly connected opening your heart with healing. Instead of living in her head and rationalizing why everything this person did was wrong, she dropped into her heart.

I have seen this miraculous healing work time and time again. I have seen families who haven't spoken in a decade or more rekindle the relationship with their loved one. The breakthroughs I have facilitated have been incredible to watch. Healing a broken relationship is the most freeing and humbling experience. It shows you unconditional love. Dropping out of the ego and the mind and into the heart is the key. It was how I healed the relationship with my father.

At the Landmark Education program, I learned a great deal about this aspect of healing. I knew I needed help after dating a series of unavailable men. The last man I dated before Landmark was a divorcee from North Carolina with two kids who lived in Alabama. He was a smoker and a manipulative person with a lot of his own unresolved issues. I broke up with him after I came to my senses that this was not the person I wanted to be with. Clearly I was a magnet for unstable, unavailable men.

What I came to discover at Landmark completely blindsided me and in retrospect it was a blessing. The Landmark Education Forum is a 45-hour weekend seminar to make peace with your past so you have the energy to powerfully move forward into the future. Everything is seen as an exciting opportunity when you can release the past. During that weekend, you are coached in a room of 100 people. You go up to the microphone and express why you are there and why you are blocked in a certain area. What I did not expect was to receive a massive breakthrough.

I went to Landmark because I didn't want to repeat the same pattern of dating loser after loser. I couldn't take the deep degree of emotional pain any longer. I didn't want to abuse my body and be so isolated from my family. When I walked up to the microphone, I choked.

"I am holding onto guilt and shame from something that happened two years ago," I said, surprising myself. *Hadn't I come here to break a pattern of dating assholes?*

"Yeah, okay. What happened?" the coach inquired. You remember Jerry, right? I talked about him earlier in the book. *All teeth, no eyes Jerry.* He was a tough-love kind of coach.

I told Jerry about getting kicked out of my house, the depths of emotional pain I felt, and the tremendous amount of courage it took for me to leave the pharmacy.

"Good. They should have kicked you out. You were 23, time to get out. Next. What's the block?" he said as I swallowed my pride.

I was shocked. He wasn't enabling me to go to the victim story. I kept going.

"Well...I keep dating asshole guys and I don't know why," I said, sobbing. "I want to break this pattern."

"Christina, my dear. Have you forgiven your parents?" he asked.

"Yes. I've done the work to release that," I said.

"Have you forgiven yourself?"

I paused and thought about that. Had I really forgiven myself for leaving the pharmacy? The automatic answer came.

"No," I replied.

"So you don't think you deserve to be happy because you left the pharmacy and now you are self-sabotaging by dating idiots and abusing your body. Is this right?"

Another hard swallow. "Yes, Jerry," I said slowly.

"What I want you to do is go call your parents and tell them how much you love them. Tell them you never wanted to be a pharmacist. Be authentic and tell them you were *in*authentic by making them believe you wanted to work there. Oh yeah, and tell them they don't need to worry about you anymore because you are taking ownership of your life."

"Damn...okay. You're right, Jerry. I need to apologize for that," I said, feeling lighter already.

During the break, I went out into the hallway and called my father.

"Dad, put Mom on speaker," I said with a tone of urgency in my voice.

"Okay, she's here. What do you need to tell us?" he asked.

"Okay, well I want to say I have not been being authentic with you.... I never wanted to be a pharmacist. I did it because unconsciously I thought I needed to in order to win your approval and have you love me. I know I have been dating asshole guys and not taking care of myself. But I want you to know that from now on you don't need to worry about me. I want us to be a family again and I love you guys so much."

"Christina, I love you too. I'm so glad you called and told us this. You are extremely mature," my father said.

My heart melted. Since when did my father open his heart and say *he loved me?*

What tends to happen in a situation from the past is that we need to separate out what really happened from our own "story." When a story is created around what happened, you suffer. We carry around stories about everything from the weather to the government to stories about the people we know on Facebook, from work, family, etc. There are payoffs and limitations with carrying a story.

For example, a story of yours might be: "My father left when I was <insert age> and that means I am not worthy of love or I cannot trust a man." When a child is young and impressionable, they draw meaning from these events. And the people around them suffer years later because the child grows up and cannot differentiate what actually happened from the story they created around it.

The situation with blaming my parents served me for so long because I didn't have to take ownership or responsibility for my own life. I was *giving my power away* to the situation and punishing myself for it. I just kept blaming that situation for any wrong choices I made in my life (financial troubles, choosing the wrong partners, my eating disorder). In reality it served me in a big way! I did not have to be responsible in my own life. It also cost me. It cut off my creativity and self-expression, it cost me my health and well-being, and it temporarily ended a real loving relationship with my family. So what was worth it in the end? Letting it all go and taking ownership of my life. Choosing to let the past be the past and drop the story.

Amazing things happen when you tell the truth, when you admit that you've been pretending things have been one way when in reality they've been another. Connections are made where they once were broken. I thought I was happy before, when in reality I was chasing things to make myself happy because I was so hurt.

Prescription to Take Your Power Back:

Take a deep inhale. Feel the feelings that are triggering you to react. Feel the anger, resentment, sadness, frustration, guilt, shame. Feel that emotion and bring it to the forefront of your consciousness.

Then release the breath and blow out all of those emotions. Acknowledge that you feel these heavy emotions.

Next, bring compassion and **forgiveness** to yourself for avoiding those feelings, holding them in, and suffering.

Accept where you are now. Be fully with the present moment.

Action steps to take your power back:

1. **Own** your part in the argument, despite the resistance that comes up. That is your ego. If you didn't care, you wouldn't be feeling so intensely about the situation. If you didn't love yourself, you wouldn't have come on this journey. Surrender to the process.

2. Think about these questions: How did you play an active role in this? How were you not being honest, truthful, or allowing yourself to "pretend" that everything was okay?

3. Write this down or speak it out loud so you are crystal clear on how you gave your power away to other people. What has holding onto this been costing you? Your health, your happiness, your self-expression, your creativity? How has it prevented you from being your true, authentic self? Keep that in your mind as your ego dissolves.

4. Place your hand over your heart and say out loud: "I promise to own my power and not give it away to others." Breathe that feeling in.

5. Write a letter or make a phone call to the person or people who you have been so readily giving your power and

energy away to. Apologize for being inauthentic with them and take ownership of the active role you played in the falling out.

*Tip: Do not go into the conversation by accusing that person of what *they did to you.* Speak clearly about yourself and come from a place of love. If you are still angry or frustrated, start the process of feeling your feelings again. Do this until you are ready to reconcile with that person.

Chapter 33: There are worse things I could do

We are so often faced with a split-moment decision and the power to choose something that serves us or does not serve us. There is a suspended moment in time where you can still alter your course of thinking to give that power away or maintain it. These boundaries are not just to be drawn or crossed with men. This is with food, sex, bosses, relatives, and even friends. Things and people that we desire yet do not serve us can tug at us the most. In Sanskrit, this is called *kama* or the desire for pleasure. Not to be confused with *karma*, kama is a desire for pleasure throughout the body; one is always seeking things to excite or please the senses.

For example, when you are eating, if you are hungry and the food tastes delicious, you can be aware of wanting to take another bite. Notice that feeling when you taste something pleasant and you want more of it. Kama can also arise from the simple joy of being alive, of admiring the beauty of nature, the pleasure that comes when you see your children safe and playing happily. These are the pleasures of life that ultimately can lead to good health, deep satisfaction, and contentment.

Then there is *dharma*, which is your life purpose. The *arta* is the means by which you reach your dharma. When kama is disconnected from dharma, desire becomes the focal point. Life becomes reduced to pleasure-seeking which cannot be sustained long-term. Addiction to physical pleasure is usually an unconscious attempt to fill the void felt when there is an absence of connection to true meaning and purpose. This is why, in some spiritual traditions, desire is seen as dangerous and difficult to manage. Indian philosophy warns against uncontrolled kama, stating that it can control you and become your master, making you its slave.

To manage desire requires training, knowledge, and experience under guidance. This leads to wisdom. By connecting kama to dharma and to your heart, you gain great emotional satisfaction and pleasure from life. You can pursue pleasure in a more balanced, healthy, and ultimately satisfying way.

On your healing journey, there may be signs that point you in the direction towards balance, health, and happiness. There may have even been several signs on the way to rock-bottom that you ignored. It's up to you to pay attention to those signs. In your heart you already know what has not served you and what desires pull at you. The key is to connect with what is underneath those desires.

We deserve to have pleasurable experiences! Of course! We are put here to be happy, to contribute and thrive! However, seeking pleasure to the extent of your demise leaves you empty, unsatisfied, and lonely. When you are connecting with the deepest part of your dharma and you align that with your kama, you will feel fulfilled.

Ultimately we are here to have love and connection with ourselves and our loved ones. To attain long-term happiness, we need to connect with our purpose. What have you always wanted to do? What do you believe is your purpose? This is the activity or thing that lights you up. Time flies and you lose track of the hours when you do this. Are you a natural writer, a photographer, an awesome mother?

Most of us have things or activities we are "good at" but do not fulfill our heart's desire. For me, that was pharmacy. I was very capable of being a perfectionist, ensuring there were no drug interactions, that the medicine I dispensed was exactly correct. But it didn't fulfill me. I knew in my heart I was not meant to be behind a counter dispensing medication to people. Something in my gut was screaming at me from the time I was 18 that this was the wrong choice. Yet I ignored and buried that voice because I didn't want to hear the hard truth.

I had a very close mentor who went through a similar process. She had been a clinical professor for 10 years at a large college before she hit rock-bottom. She suffered from frequent migraines, neck pain, hip pain, and had gained weight since she started her job. After I spoke to her about her current life situation, she expressed her dissatisfaction with her job. Being a college professor, grading papers, and attending weekly faculty meetings were not her cup of tea.

She began to meditate and go inside for the answers to get clear on her life purpose. Instead of agonizing over her migraines, she began to send that part of her love and get curious as to why it was there. After reflecting on how her health was suffering and her obvious dissatisfaction with her job, she made a bold move. She had always told me, "When you betray your own heart in exchange for money, you pay in other ways." This couldn't be more true.

Betraying your soul's calling can cost you your health, creativity, self-expression, and genuine happiness. It cost me my health for 7 years before I surrendered. You may literally be brought to your knees before you completely surrender to something larger than yourself. Your higher consciousness may have sent you messages through visions, feelings, or messages, yet you've ignored them. Your body may have told you through different signs—migraines, hip/shoulder/neck pain, an eating disorder, or a sugar addiction. You may have ignored those signs, too!

You may be like me, asking, *What is my purpose?* And at the same time doubting you could be that powerful and great. Let me tell you something—you are more capable, powerful, loving, and limitless than you ever believed possible. All you have to do is listen to yourself and go inside to find the answers.

What excuses do we give for not following our intuition or our dreams? I call these statements the "What if" statements. Whenever you start a sentence with 'What if' it usually comes from a place of fear.

- "What if I get distracted/stuck/frustrated and can't do it? I don't have enough time to pursue my dream anyway."
- "What if I go bankrupt? I can't afford to quit my job—I need it for financial security. It pays the bills."
- "What if I haven't done enough personal growth stuff to do before I can step into my power and help others? I'm damaged/broken/need healing."
- "What if no one listens/reads what I have to say anyway, what's the point?"
- "What if I fail?"
- "What if this is all just a fluffy dream and not logical/practical/rational?"

- What if I'm not worthy or deserving of this abundance?"

Do not ever let anyone tell you something is not possible. Instead of barriers, see possibilities and opportunities. Any lack of money can be attained with creativity and resourcefulness. Any lack of joy can be felt with love and found through fulfillment. And any excuse, self-doubt, or fear can be healed with the belief that you are more capable than you ever thought possible.

My mentor quit her job as a college professor after 10 years and decided to start her own coaching business. She had a baby to take care of and a husband who was not working. Yet she found her way and developed her coaching business, writing and publishing her first book (with one small child, by the way!). She wanted to show others how to "play bigger" and step into their power.

It takes extreme courage, or heart, to follow your dreams and your life purpose. Bills, children, and maintaining a roof over your head are very real. I am not telling you to quit your job today, but what I am telling you to do is to create an exit strategy. How can you transition out of your current job so that you can find time and energy to devote to what is pulling at you?

Maybe you'd like to create a small business out of your favorite hobby (baking those amazing cookies everyone loves, or creating beautiful bracelets and jewelry from home). One of the most notable hobbyists of all time is certainly Walt Disney. He turned his love of doodling and sketching into a multi-billion-dollar business that continues to thrive nearly 50 years after his death.

There is tremendous value to what you do and what you find "so easy." Other people need your services and your expertise. Your ego may fight back and say, "What could I possibly offer?" Think basic. What are you naturally good at yet get lost in? Do people come to you for support, advice, coaching? Do they love your green smoothies, shakes, cookies, or something else you make? Create a small business out of creating personalized packages for people! If you know how to create simple, healthy meals — offer that to people. Don't limit yourself and what you are capable of creating. All you need to do is create a plan for it (#1) and believe you can do it (#2).

The first part is easy because if you know your talent, gift, or dream, you can easily create packages or even seek further education in that interest if you are ambitious enough. Where we get stuck is in believing that it can't happen. Nothing will block your dream from coming to fruition more than a deep-seated negative belief.

Prescription for Examining and Releasing Fear:

So let's examine the beliefs and bust them, because they are not true! Did any of the Fear statements resonate with you? Take a blank piece of paper and pick one or two of those bullshit beliefs. Write out where those beliefs came from. Who did they come from? If you can remember, what event(s) started that belief? How did it make you feel at the time? How does it make you feel now?

_____

_____

_____

_____

_____

Now write out what has not been serving you. What has it cost you in health, happiness, time with your family, relationships with a lover? How would it cost you if you stayed in this job that does not fulfill you?

_____

_____

_____

_____

_____

The idea behind this exercise is to create emotional leverage so you have the courage to do this. Really feel these emotions that come up. Anger, sadness, regret, guilt, shame. Whatever they are, just feel them. Then take the paper and RIP IT TO SHREDS. Release all of those bullshit beliefs!

If we can bust the limiting beliefs and affect the level of the emotion, we can change the behavior. The exercise you did in writing down the limiting beliefs will get you out of the way and allow the ideas to flow. Saying it and speaking your dream to someone else will get your mind working to execute and eventually commit to it. Watch your language from now on. Only speak positively about yourself, even if it feels awkward or false and you don't _really_ believe it. What you speak you become, and the universe responds to your energy, whether you believe it or not. Change your beliefs and you change your blueprint.

For another powerful process called the Fear Inventory Process, refer to **Appendix E.** This process comes out of the 12-Step Recovery Process.

Chapter 34: Come as you are, as a friend

I began to see my eating disorder as a blessing because it called upon everything in me to heal the emotional wounds from my past. It was a constant physical reminder to manage and take care of my inner state, to connect with myself when I wanted so desperately to seek love from external sources. Most importantly, it taught me to be compassionate with myself.

In the therapy office on 12th Street, I learned to meet myself with compassion instead of judgment. For years I had fed into a vicious cycle of judgment and self-criticism, reinforcing my night-eating addiction. Judie helped me see that having love and compassion for this part of myself wasn't only lessening the addiction's hold on me, it was helping me *heal*. So much of my behavior throughout my adult life had been to strive for achievement and recognition, to be productive and successful. It didn't matter how much I weighed, how beautiful I was, whether I was a doctor of pharmacy, whether I had 1,000 friends or 2. What mattered was the amount of unconditional love I was able to give myself each and every day, despite any illusions, perceived rejections, failures, or circumstances.

Gradually I started sleeping soundly for the first time in seven years. I would wake up feeling refreshed, I was *clear-headed*. The world took on a freshness, a dream-like quality of beauty. I was unbelievably happy. After 7 years of my struggle, I was finally sleeping soundly.

For the longest time, I was hurting myself because I thought I didn't deserve love. Something from childhood made me think I was "bad" and "unworthy," but I had gained an immense awareness because of the eating disorder, and I was able to meet those thoughts with compassion.

One day on my way to a therapy appointment, I got caught in the rain. I felt free and playful as I jumped directly into deep puddles on East 12th Street on my way to Judie's office. Laughing at myself, I ran past dozens of people with their faces pressed against glass storefronts waiting for the rain to subside. I was so unbelievably happy to be alive and so grateful for the rain, the darkness I'd overcome to get to that place. That whole concept of my growth took a millisecond to process and I giggled as I hopped into 24 E 12th Street, escaping the dampness of Mother Nature. I took a picture of myself with drenched hair, raindrops abundantly seeping down my face. I took out my phone to capture the moment in a picture and all of the strangers in the lobby smiled at my naive attempt. I felt connected to myself, to people, to the world—and so I laughed at myself. I got every single one of the strangers in the lobby to smile at my outrageousness.

"Isn't life amazing?!" I wanted to scream. Because it truly was.

I had craved connection but didn't know how to get it aside from having the certainty and reliability of getting up every night to eat. Disagreements with friends or disappointments in romantic relationships felt so raw and intense that I either ended them abruptly or avoided them altogether. It was easier to be alone and free from the drama and judgments of other people. If I did attract a friendship or relationship, it was with an emotionally unavailable person or someone who needed me to take care of them. All of them were a mirror for what I harbored inside of myself at the time — unresolved pain.

The pattern was salient and similar in quality every single time. I would begin dating this ideal person, fall "in love" and get my heart wrapped in every facet of the relationship, and get high on the surge of neurotransmitters (dopamine, serotonin). Too often the word "love" was thrown around loosely in the first week or two and after a few weeks one or both of us would pull away. It took many failed relationships before realizing it wasn't just a coincidence that I was in fact attracting and accepting these unavailable men into my life. I needed to face my problems directly.

They all said the same thing — I couldn't deal with it when people disagreed with me, I was in grief about the relationship with my parents and they couldn't handle it. It messed with my head in more ways than one to hear expressions of love one minute and feel completely abandoned and emotionally distanced the next. Ultimately, abandonment was what I feared most, yet it eluded me every time.

A mentor of mine recommended a book to me called *I Need Your Love, is That True?* by Byron Katie. This book revolutionized the way I saw my behavior. We think we need love and or recognition from our parents or our significant other or our boss in order to achieve a certain feeling. We often project our own insecurities onto those people because we feel a lack. It dawned on me that I was telling certain stories to myself, especially in regard to the most important of all — the story about my father.

The story in my mind went something like this:

My father was so hard on us as kids. All we heard was, "Work hard. No money no honey." And later, Is your boyfriend a hard worker? What does he do for a living?" He was never there for us growing up. He was always working. He abandoned me when I needed help with my eating disorder and buried his head. I resent him for withholding love from me after I decided not to work for him. I resent him for giving me my eating disorder. It was his fault that I was this fucked-up. That I was this controlled and disciplined.

Byron Katie's book was designed to ask questions that would reframe your thoughts to a turnaround where you can see another viewpoint of your "story."

Question #1 was, is this all true?
Yes. I believe all of this is true. Why else would I believe it?

Question #2 was, is this absolutely true? All of the time? Always?
No. Not always. He had to work and provide for us. He did the best he could, I guess. I remember him building me a treehouse, training me for 10 years to be a pharmacist, and helping me with my homework.

What is the turnaround?
I guess I abandoned him by leaving. I see now that I was withholding love from him because I was blaming him for my eating disorder and distancing myself from him.

All of this was such a revelation. I had been projecting onto him all of my insecurities and standing in my own way. So much of my energy had been wasted trying to get him to approve of me when he was so busy just trying to provide for our family. The fact that I was his daughter was enough. In that moment I knew that I had unlocked a secret door to freeing myself from suffering not only in the relationship with my father, but in all relationships.

How much of my daily energy was spent trying to prove my worth to other people? I decided to become a detective about it instead of judging myself. I took notice of every time I tried to tell a story to make myself sound more important or have someone think a certain way about me. I began to see that I would post pictures on Facebook to have people think I was creative, sexy, intelligent, etc. A simple conversation about a drug at work was a way for me to show how smart I was. I was, in essence, manipulating people and attempting to inflate my ego.

The stories I was telling were bullshit. That type of energy was draining me. I made a clear decision to change the way I conducted myself. I started doing the opposite of what I would normally do in almost every situation. At the gym, I took a spot in the back of the class instead of the front row to avoid attention-seeking. I stayed quiet when someone at work was explaining protein benefits to a co-worker. A certain grace fell upon me; a relaxed space entered my world as I simply began observing my normal patterns of "seeking." Who was I trying to prove anything to? I had to cultivate radical self-acceptance and self-love for myself for the rest of my life before I could expect it from a partner. I was cultivating self-love…

Chapter 35: Story of my life

The world was mirroring the lessons I needed to learn and I realized that although I had been projecting my neediness for others to accept certain qualities about me, it was my job to nurture that love for myself. I had always wanted someone to see my heart, my kindness and my intelligence before my outer appearance. I devoted so much time and energy to that seeking. It was time to give that love to myself. I had been denying those core gifts for too long, suppressing them to please others and avoiding expressing them because it would make me too vulnerable.

Loving and approving of yourself takes the focus away from pleasing other people. It allows you to focus your energy in the present instead of living in the past or worrying about the future. When you are in the present moment, you imbue each activity with a quality of freshness, aliveness, and love. With this renewed energy, you attract new opportunities, stress decreases, and you find that you are more creative. It is the law of least effort, which states that all you have to do is show up and possess an energy that resonates with love and the universe works in your favor.

Love and approve of yourself. Clear your space of toxic people and situations. This will create organization in your mind, attract more loving relationships in your life, a new job and a new and better place to live, and even enable your body weight to normalize. People who love themselves and their bodies do not abuse themselves or others.

Self-approval and self-acceptance in the now are the main keys to positive changes in every area of our lives. Loving yourself begins with bringing curiosity to ourselves instead of criticism and radically accepting every aspect of who we are. Criticism locks us into the very pattern we are trying to change. Understanding and being gentle with ourselves helps us move out of it. You may have been criticizing yourself for years, and has it worked? No! Self-love is the way to healing.

Tiny miracles began taking place in my life as I became intensely connected to myself and to God. I utilized my creativity in novel ways, becoming engaged and truly listening to people when they spoke. It was effortless to find solutions to problems since I wasn't wasting energy worrying what others thought or trying to prove myself.

I had recommended a co-worker to see someone to get hypnotized for smoking cessation since it had worked wonders for me. About 2 weeks after she had been hypnotized, my co-worker's mother came into the pharmacy to see her.

My co-worker had completely stopped smoking. She could breathe again and felt healthy. We all spoke of the amazing success of the hypnosis and how proud we were of her in combating her long-standing habit.

Right before her mother left, she said, "Thank you, Christina. Because of you my daughter has her health back."

In that moment my heart expanded inside of me just like it had 10 years prior. Time froze. Tears welled up. A feeling of happiness blended with humble gratitude washed over my entire body. That *feeling* returned. *Love.* Absolute compassion and love for this woman and her daughter.

As I sat to meditate on the feeling of gratitude that night, I paused and wished I could hold onto it forever. To me, this was success. Happiness is not in the GETTING, but in the GIVING.

To have it come full-circle 10 years later was such a blessing and I sat on my couch and cried at the beauty in the gifts I had been given. I thanked God for the pain I had been put through as it was all for a reason—to serve at the highest level possible in the world. You see, often the people who have been through the most pain and learn the hardest lessons have the power to transform the culture around them. I felt absolutely blessed to have gone through my own pain and shared the ways to overcome obstacles I had struggled with.

It might have been a feeling I was continually chasing—love, acceptance, security, safety, peace, but I finally understood what feeling I needed to fulfill my purpose. It was all so intimately connected. I needed to feel and connect with my own light, my own joy to attract positive things into my life. Situations were not happening *to* me. I had the power to choose. I was in the driver's seat. I had been my own worst enemy and was now becoming my own best friend.

Chapter 36: You can't always get what you want, but sometimes you get what you need

A week later I was in the shower and had an epiphany. Don't our biggest insights always come to us in the shower? I thought about the forgiveness list I had made and drifted away to why this had all happened to me. I wondered why I never got the approval from my dad, why I had to bust my ass to get through this eating disorder.

And with a flash of insight, it all made sense. What would I have been like if everything had come easy? Would I have grown without that immense uncertainty? Would I have learned to approve of myself if my parents always had my back? I had to learn to own my power, to experience massive pain to be able to show others how to walk through theirs. I would not have had my business or the fire to break through to my purpose. I would not have had those quiet nights in solitude where I spoke to God and to my heart to understand what I was placed here to do.

I couldn't help but think that this whole path was really a gift. So many people lose faith in God or a higher power because they think, *why would God give me this disease? Why would God allow this to happen to me or my child/husband/loved one?* There is a lesson in everything, even the pain. I am not saying your pain is justified or the person who passed meant to pass. However, I am saying in each experience, there is a beautiful lesson to be learned. Maybe the lesson could be to appreciate life in the face of death. Maybe it was to connect to yourself to ease your own pain.

I came to realize that I had an idea in my mind and God had another plan. As much as I resisted, he never gave up on me. He just kept nudging me toward the place I needed to be. I was brought to my knees until I surrendered to divine will. Divine will always trumps your own will. To wake up to your full potential, you have to peel back the layers of fear, shame, and guilt, and embrace every piece of yourself.

The heart is the repository for all things beautiful. It has the elixir for the wounds to get healed, for the sins to be forgiven, and for the abundance of love to flow endlessly. In the heart there is space for self-love, love for others and strangers alike. In the depths of the heart there is space even for enemies. Just when one thinks no light can get in, compassion opens the hatch and allows the accommodation of brightness. In the heart space is where the magic, the alchemy happens.

I wanted so badly to have my message of healing reach people. Through my meditations and in the quiet moments of solitude, God spoke to me, telling me that my purpose was to tell my story. I had felt this calling since I was 18, to share both the pain and the purpose behind it. Through synchronicities with enlightened individuals and eliminating the limiting beliefs I had about myself, I began to heal.

I realized that for most of my life, I had been chasing a feeling. I chose pharmacy as a career because I wanted to feel LOVE from my father and also to CONNECT with people. I chose to dress a certain way to feel FEMININE and FREE. I recounted the peak experiences in my life: being so connected to everyone at Neptune Beach Club, visiting Albany and feeling free and boundless, dancing. I sat and meditated, feeling the bliss and joy as I recalled connecting to my patients at the pharmacy, seeing their eyes express gratitude.

The disease had manifested because I had lost touch with the core feelings when I stopped dancing, broke up with David, and moved away to college. I needed to reconnect with what made me

FEEL good in order to heal myself. I had my own prescription for healing; I just had to be still enough to receive it. Creating my health coaching business became my platform for spreading the message of self-love, healing, and joy. If other people suffered similar strife, I wanted to be the voice to inspire a radical transformation—one of true self-discovery and spiritual, emotional, and mental alchemy to transmute lead into brilliant gold.

I had suffered because I chose to give my power away, but I realized that right next to that suffering was immense joy. What if this whole roller-coaster ride was really a gift? What if my father *not* approving of me was the biggest gift of my life? It called me to step up, take my power back, and reveal my truth. I began changing my perspective. All old structures that are false eventually crumble and come to light in truth. I needed to release all of the limiting beliefs that would not serve me or the people I needed to reach.

I was meant to be a healer and a teacher, to reveal a strong message so others would not have to suffer alone. If the road had been easy, I would not have grown. If it were easy, I would not have revealed my inner radiance. What I really needed was a connection with others to heal. What I found was a connection to myself.

One day after I went back home to Copiague, I walked up to our front door and saw my father through the blinds lying on the couch watching television. I could bet he was watching the Knicks game— he loved basketball. I was so grateful for Landmark and how it helped me get clear on my awareness to take my power back. We were at a more harmonious place now.

"Hey Dad, watching the Knicks game?" I asked as I sat next to him on the couch.

"Yeah, they're playing the Bulls tonight. Looks like they're winning though." He sat up from the couch, still watching the screen.

"Where's Mom?" I asked.

"She's in the sunroom ironing," he said.

I got up to leave and say hi to my mother.

"Wait, Christina...I was going to ask you to do Reiki on my knee," he asked.

"Sure Dad, I can do that for you. Which knee is bothering you?" I was totally stunned. Since when did he believe in Reiki? He was so left-brained and pragmatic. He was a black-and-white thinker. But I didn't question it. I just scooted over next to him on the couch while the Knicks were playing. I prayed. I placed my hands gently on his left knee, the one that had the surgery a few years back. It was inflamed from years of tennis, being on his feet at the drugstore all day, and standing strong for my entire family.

My memory was flooded with seeing him at the hospital on pain medication a few years back. My dad was never vulnerable. He never had to be taken care of. I wasn't used to seeing him like that. In that moment I saw the same vulnerability.

I laid my hands on the part of his knee that was drawing the most energy. It was pulsing down his patella. "This is where the real pain is, right?" I asked, meeting his eyes.

"Yeah, right there. I put ice on it before," he said. I prayed that his pain be taken away. I prayed for the highest good of his health. I thanked God for the ability to connect with this man I admired and loved so deeply.

I had a flashback to when I was 14-year-old girl at the pharmacy so many years ago. I recalled his compassion, how he truly *felt* for the widow who had just lost her husband. As I dug deeper into that memory, I remembered he touched her arm to placate her and the subsequent heart expansion I felt. In an instant I knew why that scene had tugged at my heart. It was connection. It was touch. It was everything I had craved to be and had seen in him. I thought being a pharmacist was the *right thing to do.* At the time I had no idea it was the touch and connection that would lead me down the path I had taken. I was a health coach, a counselor for people's deepest fears and biggest successes. I was a Reiki healer, using the power of touch to help comfort and heal energy blocks. In the end, I was right where I needed to be. It just looked a little bit different than what I had imagined.

"I went to the doctor yesterday. My Ejection Fraction went up from 40 to 50," he said, speaking about the test that gauges the strength of the heart's ability to pump. A normal Ejection Fraction is over 60 and the doctor had discussed that the EF of a person with Congestive Heart Failure usually declines over time. It was very rare to see that number improve.

"Dad, that's incredible! The doctor said it wouldn't go up. I guess the daily walking and medications are helping," I replied. His heart was healing....

"How do you feel?" I asked him as I slowly detached my hands from his knee.

"Feels a lot better," he replied. He stretched the knee out and stood up. "I'm cured!" he said.

"Oh, you are so damn corny, Dad." I smiled at him. He was the same. I was the same. But something was different. And I was whole again.

Chapter 37: Shine bright like a diamond

Look around you. Are you safe? Are you supported? Can you feel the breath flowing in and out of your body? If you are reading this book then those answers should be yes. The chair or bed or floor beneath you is supporting you. Isn't it comforting to know for certain that the floor will not just fall out from under you? You are safe and supported *now*. There is no need to worry about the future or the past. The past is just a tool that has taught you how to survive, and the future is completely unknown. You do not have to be ruled by your past. You do not have to be fearful of the future because there are endless possibilities and outcomes that can manifest for you.

There is the *known* and the *unknown*, and beautiful blessings come out of the unknown. What you are used to and what creates certainty in your life is what has kept you stuck, frustrated, and safe. Human beings crave certainty because at the basic level we are wired to be safe. It is in Maslow's Hierarchy of Needs. As humans we need water, food, and shelter — all of which makes us safe. When there is an uncertainty, it feels like a threat. However, leaning into uncertainty is the way toward true growth.

I will let you in on a secret — the *known* is actually right in front of you. The present moment is the only thing that is certain and exists in the here and now. The gentle breathing of your body, the time on the clock, the beauty that comes from seeing life for exactly what it is. Take a deep breath of oxygen, of that life-force energy exchange. Now let it go and release the past, release the feelings that have held you back. Start today fresh. Start believing in yourself and your ability to create your life exactly as you'd like it to be.

What are you committed to this year? Dream big. Never filter yourself or play small. Do you want to be more loving? Do you want to quit your job and fulfill your dream? Treat your body with more love and respect? What is calling to you immediately? Commit to it, say it out loud, write it down. Speak it to the universe. Tell someone else who encourages and supports you.

Are there going to be days when you back slip into old patterns? Yes. Will there be days when you are scared shitless and want some certainty again? Be strong and have an accountability partner. Remember how *good* it feels to eat mindfully and nourish your body. Recall how amazing it felt to finally let go of that secret or that thing that was holding you back from being the radiant human being you really are.

Appendix

Appendix A: Seven Day Food Log

Day of the Week	What I ate	How I felt right after	How I felt an hour after	Mood/Energy Level
1.				
2.				
3.				
4.				
5.				
6.				
7.				

Appendix B

Release Process

Following this release process will help clear away the pain and increase your vitality, energy, and aliveness.

    1.   Sit quietly for several minutes. Think back to a memory that has come to you, maybe one you have suppressed for a while now. You know which one this is. Be gentle with yourself, offer kindness and non-judgment into your heart.

    2.   Now remember how that event felt, the images in your mind, the people, the surrounding noises, sensations, and smells. Go into that scene. Feel it. If anger, rage, sadness, or any other emotion comes up, please let it come up. Continue to breathe and focus as best you can. Maybe you were a young child, maybe it was a month ago. Offer

yourself complete compassion by placing your hand on your heart.

3.   Picture yourself seeing this scene from a bird's-eye view, almost as if you are an angel protecting yourself in the scene. Continue to offer compassion and love for yourself as you recall the memory. Remind yourself that this event was in the past and it was not your fault.

4.   Mentally go down to the child or version of you in that scene and give him/her a hug. Offer love and compassion as you do this. You may experience a softening in your heart, a dissolving of the pain. This is where healing occurs!

5.   Open your eyes. Jot down in a journal what you felt, how you feel now. If you have residual anger towards a particular person, release that anger. It is not meant to live inside of you.

Congratulations! You have just released low vibrational energies. Make sure to drink plenty of water to cleanse those toxins from your body.

Appendix C

Loving Kindness Meditation

· Put your hands over your heart to remind yourself that you are bringing not only attention, but *loving* attention, to your experience. Feel the warmth of your hands, the gentle pressure of your hands, and feel how your chest rises and falls beneath your hands with every breath.

· Now, bring to mind a person or other living being who naturally makes you smile. This could be a child, your grandmother, your cat or dog—whoever naturally brings happiness to your heart. Perhaps it's a bird outside your window. Let yourself feel what it's like to be in that being's presence. Allow yourself to enjoy the good company.

· Now, recognize how vulnerable this loved one is—just like you, subject to sickness, aging, and death. Also, this being wishes to be happy and free from suffering, just like you and every other living being. Repeat softly and gently, feeling the importance of your words:

May you be safe.
May you be peaceful.
May you be healthy.
May you live with ease.

When you notice your mind wandering, return to the words and the image of the loved one you have in mind. Savor any warm feelings that may arise.

· Now add *yourself* to your circle of good will. Put your hand over your heart and feel the warmth and gentle pressure of your hand (for just a moment or for the rest of the meditation), saying:

May you and I be safe.
May you and I be peaceful.
May you and I be healthy.
May you and I live with ease.

· Visualize your whole body in your mind's eye. Notice any stress or uneasiness that may be lingering within you, and offer kindness to yourself.

May I be safe.
May I be peaceful.
May I be healthy.
May I live with ease.

· Now take a few breaths and just rest sit quietly in your own body, savoring the good will and compassion that flows naturally from your own heart. Know that you can return to the phrases anytime you wish.

· Gently open your eyes.

I always practiced the Loving Kindness Meditation at night before I went to sleep because I had so much anxiety and fear. This meditation helps cultivate a sense of love and safety, even if you are sleeping alone. Remember, we are rarely lonely if we learn how to enjoy the company of ourselves when we are alone.

You can start with 5 minutes of guided meditation daily and work up to 30 minutes in the morning or evening for optimal benefit. Eventually you will not need a guided meditation and will be able to quiet your mind naturally. If you find you still need help and cannot focus, group meditation practice is helpful and provides great support for beginners.

The following are the plan from Dr. D'Adamo's research. Try to incorporate these small changes and see how your body responds to it. I have found in my patients that it can feel overwhelming to make a huge change all at once. Chunk down the goals into two per week to minimize that feeling of "Oh shit, I have to change my whole life." For example if you are Type A, in week one you can try to not skip breakfast and try to get more sleep. Small, manageable goals are longer lasting.

Appendix D

The Blood Type Diet
Type A:

Characteristics:

Type A's most often described themselves in ways related to the following characteristics: sensitive to the needs of others, good listeners, detail oriented, analytical, creative, and inventive.

The Diet:

To help balance cortisol levels, Dr. D'Adamo recommends that type A's limit sugar, caffeine, and alcohol. He recommends not skipping meals, especially breakfast; eating smaller, more frequent meals will also help to stabilize blood sugar levels. He also points out that the following factors are known to increase cortisol levels and increase mental exhaustion for Type A's—be aware and limit your exposure when possible.

Overall Health:

Limit your exposure to these things when possible
1. Crowds of people
2. Loud noise
3. Negative emotions

4. Smoking

5. Strong smells or perfumes

6. Too much sugar and starch

7. Overwork

8. Violent TV and movies

9. Lack of sleep

10. Extreme weather conditions (hot or cold)

The other blood types vary in characteristics, the diet to follow and how to effectively reducing stress.

Type O:

Characteristics:

Leadership, extroversion, energy and focus are among their best traits. Type O's can be powerful and productive, however, when stressed Type O's response can be one of anger, hyperactivity, and impulsivity. When Type O wiring gets crossed, as a result of a poor diet, lack of exercise, unhealthy behaviors, or elevated stress levels, Type O's are more vulnerable to negative metabolic effects, including insulin resistance, ulcers, sluggish thyroid activity, and weight gain.

The Diet:

Dr. D'Adamo does not recommend iodine supplements, rather a diet rich in saltwater fish and kelp to help regulate the thyroid gland. Type O's also have a higher level of stomach acid than the other blood types, which often results in stomach irritation and ulcers. Dr. D'Adamo recommends a licorice preparation called DGL (deglycyrrhizinated licorice) which can reduce discomfort and aid healing. DGL protects the stomach lining in addition to protecting it from stomach acids. Avoid crude licorice preparations as they contain a component of the plant that can cause elevated blood pressure. This component has been removed in DGL.

To avoid becoming overstressed, Dr. D'Adamo recommends following the Type O diet, which focuses on lean, organic meats, vegetables and fruits, and to avoid wheat and dairy, which can be triggers for digestive and health issues in Type O.

Stress Reduction:

Type O is more vulnerable to destructive behaviors when overly tired, depressed or bored. These can include gambling, sensation seeking, risk taking, substance abuse and impulsivity. Additionally, he suggests that Type O's avoid caffeine and alcohol. Caffeine can be particularly harmful because of its tendency to raise adrenaline and noradrenaline, which are already high for Type O's.

Exercise:

The Type O who exercises regularly also has a better emotional response. Dr. D'Adamo suggests that Type O's engage in regular physical activity three to four times per week. For best results, engage in aerobic activity for thirty to forty five minutes at least four times per week. If you are easily bored, choose two or three different exercises and vary your routine.

Overall Health:

In addition to exercising and eating foods that are Right for Your Type, here are a few key lifestyle strategies for Type O individuals:

    1. Develop clear plans for goals and tasks—annual, monthly, weekly, daily to avoid impulsivity.

2. Make lifestyle changes gradually, rather than trying to tackle everything at once.

3. Eat all meals, even snacks, seated at a table.

4. Chew slowly and put your fork down between bites of food.

5. Avoid making big decisions or spending money when stressed.

6. Do something physical when you feel anxious.

7. Engage in thirty to forty five minutes of aerobic exercise at least four times per week.

8. When you crave a pleasure releasing-substance (alcohol, tobacco, sugar), do something physical.

Type B:

Characteristics:
Subjective, easygoing, creative, original, and flexible. The primary challenges that can get in the way of optimum health for Type B include a tendency to produce higher than normal cortisol levels in situations to stress; sensitivity to the B specific lectins in select foods, resulting in inflammation and greater risk for developing Syndrome X; susceptibility to slow growing, lingering viruses — such as those for MS, CFS, and lupus; and a vulnerability to autoimmune diseases.

The Diet:
For Type B's the biggest factors in weight gain are corn, wheat, buckwheat, lentils, tomatoes, peanuts and sesame seeds. Each of these foods affect the efficiency of your metabolic process, resulting

in fatigue, fluid retention, and hypoglycemia—a severe drop in blood sugar after eating a meal. When you eliminate these foods and begin eating a diet that is right for your type, you blood sugar levels should remain normal after meals. Another very common food that Type Bs should avoid is chicken. Chicken contains a Blood Type B agglutinating lectin in its muscle tissue. Although chicken is a lean meat, the issue is the power of an agglutinating lectin attacking your bloodstream and the potential for it to lead to strokes and immune disorders. Dr. D'Adamo suggests that you wean yourself away from chicken and replace them with highly beneficial foods such as goat, lamb, mutton, rabbit and venison. Other foods that encourage weight loss are green vegetables, eggs, beneficial meats, and low-fat dairy. When the toxic foods are avoided and replaced with beneficial foods, Blood Type B's are very successful in controlling their weight.

Stress Reduction:

When it comes to hormones, type B is closer to type A, producing somewhat higher levels of cortisol. When a Type B is out of balance, this manifests in overreaction to stress, difficulty in recovering from stress, disrupted sleep patterns, daytime brain fog, disruptive to GI friendly bacteria and suppresses immune function. This leads to increased risks for depression, insulin resistance, hypothyroidism, and high stress can further exacerbate virtually all health challenges.

Dr. D'Adamo has observed that Type B's have a wonderful gift to be able to gain physiological relief from stress and maintain emotional balance through the utilization of mental processes such as visualization and meditation.

Exercise:

To maintain the mind/body balance that is unique to Type B's, Dr. D'Adamo recommends that you choose physical exercise that challenges your mind as well as your body. Type B's need to balance meditative activities with more intense physical exercise. Excellent forms of exercise for Type B's include tennis, martial arts, cycling, hiking, and golf.

Overall Health:

1.   Visualization is a powerful technique for Type B's. If you can visualize it, you can achieve it.

2.   Find healthy ways to express your nonconformist side.

3.   Spend at least twenty minutes a day involved in some creative task that requires your complete attention.

4.   Go to bed no later than 11:00pm and sleep for eight hours or more. It is essential for B's to maintain their circadian rhythm.

5.   Use meditation to relax during breaks.

6.   Engage in a community, neighborhood or other group activity that gives you a meaningful connection to a group. Type B's are natural born networkers.

7.   Be spontaneous.

As they age, Type B's have a tendency to suffer memory loss and have decreased mental acuity. Stay sharp by doing tasks that require concentration, such as crossword puzzles or learn a new skill or language

Type ABO:

Characteristics:
Type AB has a unique chameleon like quality—depending on the circumstances, this blood type can appropriate the characteristics of each of the other blood types. Type AB is sometimes A-like, sometimes B-like, and sometimes a fusion of both. Type AB often receives mixed messages about emotional health. While you tend to be drawn to other people and are friendly and trusting, there is a side of you that feels alienated from the larger community. At your best, you are intuitive and spiritual, with an ability to look beyond the rigid confines of society. You are passionate in your beliefs, but you also want to be liked by others and this can create conflicts.

The Diet:
Type AB has Type A's low stomach acid, however they also have Type B's adaptation to meats. Therefore, you lack enough stomach acid to metabolize them efficiently and the meat you eat tends to get stored as fat. Your Type B propensities cause the same insulin reaction as Type B when you eat lima beans, corn, buckwheat, or sesame seeds.

Type AB should avoid caffeine and alcohol, especially when you're in stressful situations. Dr. D'Adamo recommends that Type

AB focus on foods such as tofu, seafood, dairy and green vegetables if you are trying to lose weight. There is a wide variety of seafood for Type AB, and it is an excellent source of protein for Type AB. A few highly beneficial fish are mahi-mahi, red snapper, salmon, sardines, and tuna. Some dairy is also beneficial for Type AB— especially cultured dairy such as Yogurt and kefir. Dr. D'Adamo also recommends smaller, more frequent meals, as they will counteract digestive problems caused by inadequate stomach acid and peptic enzymes.

Your stomach initiates the digestive process with a combination of digestive secretions, and the muscular contractions that mix food with them. When you have low levels of digestive secretions, food tends to stay in the stomach longer. He also suggests that Type AB pay attention to combining certain foods. For example, you'll digest and metabolize foods more efficiently if you avoid eating starches and proteins in the same meal.

Stress Reduction/Exercise:
Your greatest danger is the tendency to internalize your emotions, especially anger and hostility, which is much more damaging to your health than externalizing it. Exercise plays a critical component in stress reduction and maintaining a healthy emotional balance for Type AB. Dr. D'Adamo recommends a combination of both calming activities and more intense physical exercise to help maintain an optimal balance. For example, three days of aerobic exercise such as running or biking and two days of calming exercise such as yoga or *tai chi*.

Overall Health:

1. Cultivate your social nature in welcoming environments. Avoid situations that are highly competitive.

2. Avoid ritualistic thinking and fixating on issues, especially those you can't control or influence.

3. Develop a clear plan for goals and tasks — annually, monthly, weekly, daily — to avoid rushing.

4. Make lifestyle changes gradually, rather than trying to tackle everything at once.

5. Engage in forty-five to sixty minutes of aerobic exercise at least twice a week. Balanced by daily stretching, meditation, or yoga.

6. Engage in a community, neighborhood or other group activity that gives you a meaningful connection to a group.

7. Practice visualization techniques daily.

8. Also carve out time alone. Have at least one sport, hobby, or activity that you perform independently of others.

It sounds like all of us could benefit from any one of these lists! So much of nutrition is trial and error and making sure you are doing what is best for YOU. For more information about Dr. D'Adamo's Blood Type Diet, visit www.dadamo.com

Remember, you have an opportunity to nourish your body three times a day, or in 5 to 6 small meals a day. That is all up to you and your bioindividuality. Whatever feels right to you and your body, do it!

Appendix E

Fear Inventory Instructions

This practice is meant to help you notice and then clear out the fear that is stuck in your body and mind, keeping you at a distance from yourself and the world. For the purposes of this exercise, we state that no fear is real. Instead, we say that all fear is "False Evidence Appearing Real," and therefore can be released and let go without any consequences other than a welcome experience of deep relief.

Step 1. Choose a "Higher Power" to address the inventory to (God, the Universe, my Higher Self — anything that is bigger than little old you).

Step 2. Choose a resentment to inventory. A resentment, for the purposes of this exercise, is defined as a person, event, or situation that is being "re-sent" through your mind, over and over. It might be your mother, your job, your health, your dog, a conversation you had with your co-worker, or some aspect of yourself that is holding you back.

Step 3. Start writing:

God, I am resentful at _____ because I have fear that...
  I have fear that...
  I have fear that...
  I have fear that...
  I have fear that...
  I have fear that...

Example: God, I am resentful at my partner because I have fear that I am not good enough for him. I have fear that I chose him for the wrong reasons. I have fear that I am mean. I have fear I secretly want him to die. I have fear that if he dies I will be left alone....

Write out the complete sentence including "I have fear that..." each and every time. Do not skip it.

Remember the fears are about actions YOU are responsible for. When in doubt, use one of these stems: "I have fear that I will choose to..." or "I have fear that I secretly want to..." or "I have fear that I sabotage myself by..." or "I have fear that I will pretend that..." or "I have fear that I choose not to see that..."

Step 4. Keep writing fears until you feel complete. They will likely veer very quickly away from the original resentment; let it go. The resentment is a point of entry for a lot of other fears. Some people write pages and pages of fears under one resentment.

Step 5. Once you are done with that resentment, move on to the next. "God, I am resentful at _____ because I have fear that....I have fear that....I have fear that...."

Keep going until that resentment is complete. Do another resentment, and keep doing new resentments until you feel complete (or run out of time).

Step 6. Once you are finished, write this prayer:

"God (or whoever you've been addressing the inventory to), I ask you to remove these fears. I pray only for knowledge of your will for us and the power to carry it out. For me and _____, _____, _____, and _____."

Fill in the blanks with the people/situations/objects that you used as resentments in the inventory.

Appendix F: List of High and Low Vibrational Foods

Examples of High Vibrational Foods:

-Wheatgrass

-Fresh certified organic fruit and vegetables food (especially greens and living grains such as sprouts)

-Natural supplements e.g. spirulina

-Herbal Teas

-Herbs and spices

-Pure or filtered water

-Olive oil

-Nuts and seeds

-Fermented Foods

-Raw chocolate (cacao nuts or their butters)

-Raw honey & maple syrup

-Legumes

-Grains such as couscous, kamut, buckwheat, brown rice, amaranth, spelt and barley

What to expect from eating high vibrational foods:

When you initially start to eat these foods, you may experience the release of trapped emotions and changes in energy levels. Fatigue, headache or nausea may occur because of the body's natural detoxification process. Make sure you are drinking plenty of water and resting your body. Be gentle with yourself, especially if you are used to eating processed foods or low vibrational foods (see list below.) The way you eat will influence your mood and elevate your outlook on life because your vibrational energy is lifted.

It may also be helpful to write in your journal how you feel before and after you start incorporating these high vibrational foods in order to see the clear difference in energy state, mental clarity and how your body feels.

Examples of Low Vibrational Foods:
-Animal meat is the densest of all foods because it contains the karma and anger/fear energies of the animal before it was killed. This is especially true if the animal was not treated properly and was fed hormones.

-Genetically modified (GMO) food, and conventional food that has been treated with chemicals and pesticides

-White rice and flours

-Sugars, Artificial Sweeteners

-Coffee/Caffeinated Beverages

-Alcohol

-Processed, packaged, canned and fast foods

-Unhealthy oils e.g. canola, cottonseed, margarine, lard and vegetable oils

-Frozen foods

-Pasteurized cows' milk, yogurt, and cheese

-Cooked foods, deep-fried foods, and microwaved food

References

"Overdose Death Rates." *Infographics*. National Institutes of Health, n.d. Web.

"Eat Right 4 Your Type®." *Welcome to the Blood Type Diet*. N.p., n.d. Web.

"Successful Prevention of Tardive Dyskinesia: A 20-year Study of 64,000 patients." *Journal of Orthomolecular Psychiatry*. January 1991.

Gonzales R, Steiner JF, Sande MA. Antibiotic prescribing for adults with colds, upper respiratory tract infections, and bronchitis by ambulatory care physicians. *Journal of the American Medical Association* Sep 17, 1997; 278: 901 - 904.

Kaptchuk, T.J., Kelly, J.M., Conboy, L.A., Davis, R.B., Kerr, C.E., Jacobsen, E.E., Kirsch, I., Schyner, R.N., Nam, B.H., et al, . (2008). Components of placebo effect: randomised controlled trial in patients with irritable bowel syndrome. BMJ, online first(April 7), 1-8.

Katie, Byron, and Michael Katz. *I Need Your Love-- Is That True?: How to Stop Seeking Love, Approval, and Appreciation and Start Finding Them Instead*. New York: Three Rivers, 2005. Print.

Robbins, Anthony. *Unleash the Power Within*. N.p.: Nightingale Conant, 2000. Print.

Small DM, Jones-Gotman M, Dagher A: Feeding-induced dopamine release in dorsal striatum correlates with meal pleasantness ratings in healthy human volunteers. *Neuroimage* 2003;19:1709-1715.

Virtue, Doreen. *Losing Your Pounds of Pain: Breaking the Link between Abuse, Stress, and Overeating*. Carlsbad, CA: Hay House, 2002. Print.

About the Author

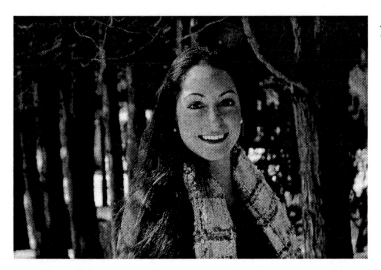

Dr.

Christina Tarantola is the Founder of NutriGlo Consulting, a health coaching company that encourages and serves soulful health and wellness inspiration. Dr. Christina is a Licensed Pharmacist, Certified Health Coach, and Reiki Healer. She incorporates nutrition/lifestyle modification, energy healing, and stress-reduction techniques into her personalized healing approach.

Dr. Christina's mission is to help reconnect people with the love, radiance, and energy within them. When you begin to Reveal Your Inner Radiance, you naturally uncover your joy and fulfillment, which is what we all seek. This journey begins within and creates a powerful domino effect, ultimately making a positive impact on our world.